Herbert Viefhues (Ed.)

Medical Manpower in the European Community

With 18 Figures and 74 Tables

Springer-Verlag
Berlin Heidelberg New York
London Paris Tokyo

Prof. Dr. Herbert Viefhues
Institut für Sozialmedizin
Ruhr-Universität Bochum
Postfach 102148, D-4630 Bochum

ISBN 978-3-540-18733-2 ISBN 978-3-642-87464-2 (eBook)
DOI 10.1007/978-3-642-87464-2

Library of Congress Cataloging-in-Publication Data
Medical manpower in the European community/Herbert Viefhues (Ed.).
p. cm.
Contents: Denmark/J. P. Steensen - Medical manpower in France / Bui Dang Ha Doan - Federal Republic of Germany / J. F. V. Deneke - Greece / A. Kalandici and A. Ritsatakis - Ireland / A. Walsh - Italy / P. L. Morosini - United Kingdom / S. Birch and A. Maynard - Problems related to future medical demography in the European community / A. Ritsatakis.

1. Medical personnel - European Economic Community countries - Statistics.
2. European Economic Community countries - Statistics, Medical.
RA410.9.E85M43 1988 331.11'9161'094 - dc 19 88-1593

Foreword

The aim of this book is to provide a snapshot of medical manpower in each of the member countries of the European Community, an exhausting untertaking in view of the problems associated with the collection of data. Complications arise in trying to apply a reasonably uniform definition for doctors in employment; some women doctors work only part-time, some doctors fill two positions, and others are theoretically retired but continue to work. Assessment of the number of students training to become doctors is confounded by differences in university curricula and in pass rates for individual examinations, and, of course, by the changing demography of each country. Information on the number of nurses, technologists, and others working within the health service might have supplied some explanation for the striking disparities in the number of doctors employed per head of population between the European countries, but such international comparisons are undermined by differences in medical practice.

Several of the member countries are striving to develop policies concerning the use of medically qualified manpower and to calculate their requirements. This is an exceedingly difficult task since medical practice and lay expectations of medical care are fluid. The number of qualified doctors practising today may be completely inappropriate in 20 years' time if dramatic changes in treatment or investigation are introduced or if patients demand lengthier consultations with their doctors. Medical and health service policies differ fundamentally between the member countries, and this will clearly influence projection for manpower requirements.

The authors were charged with supplying a description of medical manpower in the European Community and not with providing a critique of manpower policies within each country. They are to be congratulated on the mammoth task involved in the assembly of these data, which, hopefully, will enable future manpower analyses to be put into prespective.

E. Bennet

Foreword

The Epidemiology and Social Medicine panel comprises representatives of the Scientific Associations of Social Medicine and Epidemiology within the European Community. Its function is to advise the Commision on policy issues and to initiate the collection of information relevant to the formulation of policy on a Community-wide basis.

The development of a single medical manpower policy within the Community is a formidable and contentious responsibility. It must contend with the variation not only in the number of medical students each member country trains, but also in the training curriculum employed and in the pattern of medical practice. Furthermore, the nature of medical training and the delivery of health services have changed substantially over the past 40 years, and the chief handicap facing the Commission is the paucity of information regarding the medical training programmes and medical manpower policies in operation in member countries.

The work reported in this book attempts to describe the current manpower policies of member countries. As chairman of the panel, I am most grateful to Professor Viefhues for the enormous amount of work that he and his colleagues have undertaken and which has served a fundamental purpose – plans for future policy can now be considered with reference to the contemporary picture.

Walter W. Holland

Contents

List of Authors

Professor Herbert Viefhues MD DMSA (Edin.)
Abteilung für Sozialmedizin and Epidemiologie
Ruhr-Universität Bochum
Stiepeler Straße 129, 4630 Bochum 1, FRG

Dr. E.A. Bennett
Director
Commission of the European Communities
Bâtiment Jean Monnet, Plateau du Kirchberg, Luxembourg

Professor W.W. Holland MD FRCGP FRCP FFCM
Department of Community Medicine
University of London
St. Thomas's Campus, London, SE1 7EH, Great Britain

Dr. Stephen Birch
Department of Community Medicine
University of Sheffield
Beech Hill Road
Sheffield S10 2TN, Great Britain

Dr. Bui Dang Ha Doan
Directeur
Centre de Sociologie et de Démographie Médicales
60, Bld de Latour-Maubourg, 75007 Paris, France

Professor D. Deliège
Faculté de Médecine
Université Catholeque de Louvain
Clos Chapelle aux Champs 30.41, 1200 Bruxelles, Belgium

Professor J.F. Volrad Deneke MD
Axenfeldstraße 16, 5300 Bonn-Bad Godesberg, FRG

Anna Kalandidi MD
Assistant Professor
Department of Hygiene and Epidemiology
School of Medicine, University of Athens
Athens (609) Goudi, Greece

Professor Alan Maynard
Director
Centre for Health Economics, University of York
York, Y01 5DD, Great Britain

Professor Peer Luigi Morosini MD
Istituto Superiore di Sanita
Laboratorio di Epidemiologia e Biostatistica
Viale Regina Elena, 299, 00161 Roma-Nomentano, Italy

Anna Ritsatakis
Department of Hygiene and Epidemiology
School of Medicine, University of Athens
Athens (609) Goudi, Greece

Jens Peter Steensen MD
Danish Hospital Institute
Nyropsgade 18, 1602 Copenhagen, Denmark

Dr. Alphonsus Walsh
Chief Medical Officer
Department of Health
Custom House, Dublin 1, Ireland

Introduction

H. Viefhues

1 Medical Manpower – Present Situation in the European Economic Community

The most important results of this study can be summarized in the following points:

The number of doctors in the European Economic Community (EEC) has almost doubled over the last 20 years. The general opinion is that supply will exceed demand, if the present number of doctors increases to the same extent as before, and that demand will still be exceeded even if there is a slight increase.

This leads to the question of the demand for doctors[1], which is a very crucial point. The general demand is governed by the following three factors.

1. The demographic factor, i.e. whether the population is increasing or decreasing. It is generally estimated that the overall population figure will fall, the number of elderly people (> 65 years) will increase and the proportion of the very young (< 1 year) will decrease. Futhermore, the general morbidity of the elderly (> 65 years) is 4 times as high as within the under 30 group and the general morbidity of women is 29% higher than that of men. We have to take these ratios into consideration when we try to assess the demand for doctors.
2. Socio-economic factors. The growth of urbanization (morbidity in cities with more than 100 000 inhibitants is 50% higher than in small communities) is such that a concentration of a maximum of 50% of the population in cities with over 100 000 inhabitants equals a growth in demand of about 8%.
   In the United States, the number of doctor–patient contacts depends on the patient's educational level (which corresponds to his income), and the same pattern of health behaviour is found in the Federal Republic of Germany, for example, where a free insurance scheme covers 98% of the population. It is estimated that a maximum upgrading of the educational level would raise the demand for doctors by about 12%. Since

1 The estimations of medical demand given here are based on those contained in *Hochschulabsolventen im Beruf – Ausbildungsbedarf für Mediziner bis zum Jahr 2000.* McKinsey & Co. Inc., Munich, 1974.

the demographically caused increase in demand will not exceed 8%, the socio-economic factor may entail an increase of 15% in the next 20 years.

3. Development in the progress of medical case. The most intensive factors in raising the demand will lie not so much in the curative sector of medicine as in the preventive one (primary and secondary prevention, e.g. early detection and treatment of disease). In the same way as the preventive sector, occupational health will expand and a growing proportion of doctors may work full-time in this field.
   Progress in curative medicine and development of psychiatric care (including psychotherapy) will perhaps create a growing demand of 5%–15%, so that as a result of the advances in medicine, these may represent an overall growth of 20%-30%.
   Even if one adds together all the above-mentioned factors in an optimistic spirit, one will still be led to predict a growth in demand of 50%–60% within the next 20 years, compared with an increase of 100% in the number of doctors, if it is assumed that the present growth will continue.

The composition of the medical profession as a social group will be less coherent than before. Doctors as a group with high-group cohesion will experience conflicts between the generations, because the profession is constantly becoming younger, and between the sexes, because the number of women in the profession is constantly growing. These conflicts will increase, as will competition. As the number of doctors grows and the income of each physician decreases, the in-group prestige will decline.

The geographical distribution of doctors is unequal in all countries. Regions with a high density of physicians contrast with those of lower density. Doctors in some countries congregate in lager cities, around universities, in regions with greater recreational facilities, better climatic conditions, etc. But this applies mostly to highly specialized physicians and not to general practitioners (GPs), but even among specialists the tendency to settle in formerly neglected or in unattractive regions is constantly growing. However, these geographical inequalities will not be so important in the future because as a result of the growing density of the transport and communications network, "remote" regions will no longer exist, and there will be access to practically every medical speciality. Especially within the densly populated countries of the EEC (e.g. Netherlands, Belgium, Federal Republic of Germany), almost every medical facility is available to everyone. However, it has to be admitted that lack of an adequate transport and communications network in some countries creates areas with too few doctors, with the result that there is little room for an additional supply of medical manpower.

Within the medical profession *the division of labour* is traditionally quite different between the United Kingdom and the continental European countries, and within the latter countries themselves. The same is true of the demarcation between the activities of doctors and those of ancillary services. It is therefore virtually impossible to make generalizations about the redistribution of tasks in future years and how this may lead to a greater demand for doctors. It has to be borne in mind, moreover, that medicine is practised in different national and therefore cultural settings. Indeed, the socio-cultural setting may have hitherto prevented a "migration" of the "medical nations" from taking place.

An up-grading of the position of GPs is noticeable in all countries, but their number is increasing in some countries and falling in others, compared with the number of specialists. In some countries, the GP is increasingly being replaced by the specialist in internal medicine, who takes over the tasks of a family doctor in the coordination and integration of the work of the specialists.

All the above observations – only a few of the highlights of the medical scene in the EEC – have to be kept in mind when dealing with doctor-inhabitants ratios or similar statistics which sometimes lead not only to miscalculations but also to misinterpretations.

2 Planning and Regulation of Medical Manpower

Except in countries with national health services, there is little or no health planning in most EEC countries and therefore little or no medical manpower planning. In most of those countries, there are only a few legal possibilities which allow the State or the self-governing medical profession to intervene with regard to the freedom of the individual to choose his vocation and to practise it.

Such intervention is forbidden under some constitutions. The authorities are therefore unable directly to restrict the number of doctors and have recourse instead to indirect means. However, the use of such means is monitored by the public, and media and the courts, and the authorities are always required to indicate that they have exhausted all possibilities of avoiding public intervention.

Indirect influences on medical demography are:

1. Limited access to medical schools (*numerus clausus*). (Here we have to distinguish between countries in which the final examination taken during secondary education of a certain level gives the right of access to tertiary education and those countries in which this examination indicates only that the student is qualified to enter a university.)
2. Limited access to further training (specialists, GPs, etc.) and relevant examinations
3. Limited access to the health care institutions (contracts with national health services, compulsory health insurance schemes, etc.)

While access to medical schools depends on students' abilities, the further training leading to specialist or GP examinations depends to a lesser extent on practice training positions and to a greater extent on hospital training positions. Both, but especially the latter, are related to hospital capacities. At the same time, the number of doctors was and is greatly increasing, the costs of the different national health services are soaring and all EEC countries are doing their utmost to restrict health service costs. However, as a result of this, the numer of training posts in hospitals is diminishing and the chances of delays in training and of bottle-necks are increased as is the amount of unpaid or underpaid work by trainees. The decreasing profitability of practices, whether in the case of single-handed practioners or doctors in group practice, will certainly not be an incentive to go into practice, and as a result of the reduction in the number of hospital beds, there is only a limited possibility of lifelong salaried posts in hospitals. It is not surprising therefore, that unemployed doctors are now to be found in almost all EEC countries.

Even the above-mentioned examples of indirect restrictions on medical manpower are rarely, if ever, the same from one EEC country to another; sometimes, they are not even consistent within individual countries.

3 Necessary Steps for Intervention by the European Economic Community

Since the number of doctors will exceed the demand for medical care over the next 20 years, it is necessary to intervene at the level of the EEC in view of the freedom enjoyed by doctors who are nationals of EEC countries to practise in any country in the Community.

The following steps are suggested:

1. Unifying the criteria for access to medical schools, such criteria to be liberal but nevertheless restrictive, and to ensure the high quality of students
2. Establishing general models of intervention, with the aim of channeling the existing abundance of doctors and planning for the future in order to avoid further abundance
3. Indicating in those models a wide range of possibilities to enable each country to make its own way according to its traditions and existing legislation

The following contributions are studies of six EEC member countries and they reveal the dilemma concerning medical manpower in the Community.

Belgium

D. Deliège

Introduction

This report provides a detailed description of the position of medical doctors in Belgium, of existing "manpower" policies and of alternatives in the light of relevant research and studies.

Chapter 1 is devoted to an overview of the supply of qualified medical personnel, both now and in the future, examining whether they are all active potential competitors on the health-care market and whether they are distributed evenly over the whole country.

Chapter 2 examines those mechanisms already in existence for controlling the supply: effective obstacles and direct or indirect regulation and persuasion, e.g. through the supply of information.

Chapter 3 covers research to underpin the development of a rational policy in this field and the ensuring suggestions on action to be taken. The following aspects are covered:

- Models identifying the links between supply, demand and other socio-economic parameters
- Various interpretations of the concept of 'needs'
- Forecasts concerning the various constituents of the system, not only the available medical manpower but also the extent to which this supply is exploited and under what conditions (workload, daily schedule, income, etc.)
- Proposed action, comprising (a) the use to be made of existing medical staff – e.g. new roles, more equal distribution of work and territory, limitations on expenditures and on the number of patients seen by any one individual as alternatives to limiting access to the profession or to a specialization; and (b) an examination of the advisability of limiting access to medical schools in order to limit available medical manpower from 1990 onwards.

1 The Extent of Supply

We now know rather accurately how many doctors there are in Belgium, regular data on this being available from a number of sources (Sect. 1.1). A detailed analysis has been made of the relevant structures and of changes within them, revealing trends associated with the recent huge increase in numbers. In particular, it has been possible to make a fundamental distinction between the number of graduates and the number of doctors treating patients. The second category is the only valid basis for analyses of the health system and reflects the real potential competition facing young graduates (Sect. 1.2). A study was also made of the geographical distribution of practitioners, revealing amazing disparities; these varied, depending on whether the doctors concerned were GPs or specialists, between the north and south of the country, between smaller geographical units within these regions (arrondissements), between urban and rural areas, etc. (Sect. 1.3).

Finally, forecasts of the situation in both 1990 and 2000 indicated that the likely number of inhabitants per graduate would be below 250. Due attention has been paid to the significance and relevance of this ratio (Sect. 1.4).

1.1 Sources of Information

A large number of indexes or lists classify doctors on the basis of either address or qualifications, depending on the specific aims of the body providing the data.[1] However, complete and regular coverage is provided by only four sources:

[1] Footnote see page 42.

- The Ministry of Health – in the *Annuaires statistiques de La Santé Publique*
- The *Institut National d'Assurance Maladie-Invalidite* – in its *Rapports généraux*
- In publications by the *Socio-Economie de la Santé* Research Unit of the University of Louvain
- In the case of specialists, in special editions of the *'Cahiers – GBS'* issued by the *Groupement Belge des Spécialistes*

1.2 Overview: Existing Structures and Past Trends

1.2.1 Total Number of Physicians

The number of graduates has tripled in the past 30 years, although the population has increased by only 14%. There has been particularly strong growth since the 1970s, although population growth remained almost static, increasing by only 1.6% in 10 years. Moreover, by the end of 1984 the number of inhabitants per doctor had fallen to 330 (Table 1). This rough indicator is misleading, however, as will be shown later on.

1.2.2 Demographic Structure

1.2.2.1 An Increasingly Young Profession

The profession is becoming increasingly youthful as a result of its accelerated growth. Younger doctors comprise a growing proportion of the total number of graduates and are entering a market in which there are only few older doctors that they are assumed to be replacing.

As is shown in Table 2, 40% of doctors in 1982 were less than 35 years of age, while only 9% were over 65 and 12% were aged between 55 and 64. Overall, the average age was 42 years.

1.2.2.2 More Women in the Profession

It is apparent just from Table 2 that more women are taking up medicine. They are much younger than the men, 62% being less than 35 years of age and over 80% less than 45. For their male colleagues the respective figures are only 35% and 58%.

The increasing proportion of women is even more evident from Table 3, which shows the proportion of women as a percentage of all doctors within given age brackets. This

---

1 – *Listes des personnes habilitées à exercer l'Art de Guérir* (approved medical practitioners), published annually by the provincial medical authorities
- The register of medical practitioners in each province
- *Annuaire des médecins spécialistes,* published by the *Institute National d'Assurance Maladie-Invalidité*
- *Annuaire de la Santé Publique* (published by Bodden et Dechy, a private advertising company)
- Telephone directories
- Lists compiled by the *Groupement Belge des Médecins-Spécialistes*

Table 1. Trends in the total number of doctors

At year's end	Number of doctors Total	Index	Number of doctors/ 10 000 people	Number of people/ doctor
1951	8 685	100	9.98	1 002
1955	9 937	114	11.17	895
1960	11 730	135	12.75	784
1965	13 793	159	14.52	689
1971	14 887	171	15.43	648
1975	18 506	213	18.86	530
1980	24 536	282	24.90	402
1983	27 631	318	28.00	357
1985	29 799	343	30.23	331

Source: *L'offre médicale et paramédicale en Belgique.* Ministry of Social Affairs and University of Louvain (1983) p. 50.

Table 2. Breakdown of medical manpower by age and sex (end of 1982)

Age	Number of doctors		Doctors practising medicine at least occasionally			
			Men		Women	
	Total	%	Total	%	Total	%
< 35	10 737	40.4	7 294	35.1	2 501	62.1
35–44	5 754	21.6	4 787	23.0	779	19.3
45–54	4 549	17.1	4 018	19.3	415	10.3
55–64	3 217	12.1	2 843	13.7	238	5.9
65 +	2 336	8.8	1 860	8.9	96	2.4
	26 593		20 802		4 029	

Source: *L'offre médicale et paramédicale en Belgique, une analyse.* Ministry of Social Affairs (1983), p.60.

trend can be confirmed from other sources: 27.6% of graduates doing specialized training are women, while women comprise 40% of first-year medical students.

The increased involvement of women helps to boost the total number of graduates coming onto the market. Over the past decade, 15% of the increase was due to a growing share of women, but no less than 84% of the increase was due to other factors.

1.2.3 Non-active and Non-practising Graduates

By no means are all graduates working, and many who are have found employment elsewhere than in public health care. The 'market' significance of a graduate may differ widely in terms of the competition he represents for colleagues already practising. This is an important point which must be taken into account when making forecasts or when drawing up regional statistics designed to help young doctors decide where to establish a practice.

Table 3. Proportion of women in particular age-groups as a percentage of all those practising medicine, even occasionally

Age	Proportion of women
Over 65	4.9
55–65	7.7
45–55	9.4
35–45	14.0
Less than 35	25.5

Source: *L'offre médicale et paramédicale en Belgique, une analyse.* Ministry of Social Affairs (1983), p.60.

1.2.3.1 Activity Rates

A number of medical graduates are not currently employed. This may be because they have retired, because they never entered the employment market or because they have left it for a period, for example to raise young children. Others may be working, but in positions that cannot be traced from available sources, e.g. in the pharmaceutical industry, for companies dealing in medical equipment, or at other jobs less obviously linked with their qualifications. On this basis, they are regarded as 'non-active' for the purpose of our statistics, in that they are not carrying out health care, preventive medicine or research in Belgium. There is a growing proportion of such 'non-active' graduates, increasing from 4.6% of all graduates in 1979 to 10% in 1985. One possible explanation is that this trend is solely the result of demographic changes – with more doctors in a certain age-group retiring and a greater number of women in the profession (who often spend some time away raising children) resulting in an overall drop in the activity rate.

Although these aspects have contributed slightly to the decreasing activity rate, they cannot explain the drop entirely, since there is an increased tendency not to make use of qualifications in all age classes and among both sexes. In the case of older doctors, it might be assumed that they are retiring earlier in response to a general change in attitudes and better pension conditions. In other age groups, the explanation is harder to find as the decrease contradicts some general sociological trends – particularly the greater involvement of women in the work force. A plausible but not verified hypothesis is that some graduates have not been able to find work, especially in the field of health care, because of the increasing competition in the field. It would thus be a reliable indicator of the prevalent glut.

1.2.3.2 Health Care

The provincial medical authorities maintain a separate classification for graduates without any 'clinical practice', i.e. those not carrying out health care either within their own practice or in a hospital. This group includes not only those graduates who are completely 'non-active' but also those whose work requires no contact with patients. They comprise an increasing proportion of all graduates, rising from 5.6% to 6.6% between 1976 and 1982, particularly among GPs, where they comprise 12% of the total as against only 2.5% of specialists and no trainee-specialists whatever. The remaining doctors, those listed as having a 'clinical practice', comprise all graduates likely to come into contact with patients, even if only on a part-time basis or occasionally. This total figure does not, therefore, reflect the potential medical care actually available to patients.

1.2.3.3 The Various Type of Activity

In order to get a better picture of what is happening in practice, it would seem advisable to make a breakdown of the various activities carried out by graduates and then to calculate new totals for each activity on the basis of the time devoted to it. This would then allow a 'whole-time equivalent' (WTE) figure to be given for the various activities carried out by medical practitioners. Ideally, this would best be done by organizing regular detailed surveys, with doctors being required to specify how they allocate their time on the basis of a list of activities drawn up beforehand. Alternatively, a pragmatic approach could be used, applying specific techniques of data collection, recording and analysis (see Appendix 1) to study the phenomenon.

This method differs from the survey mainly in that it gives an equal weight to the different kinds of activity in inverse proportion to the number of locations at which each graduate is listed as working, in other words, not taking into account the time actually spent on each activity. While this hypothesis is clearly incorrect at an individual level, it is acceptable at a regional or a national one – the corollary being that occasional health care work on the part of some graduates is balanced by other graduates occasionally carrying out other types of work. Put more simply, whatever the approach adopted, a doctor with administrative responsibilities, but also running his own part-time practice, and a doctor devoting most of his time to the practice, but also acting twice a week as a consultant in preventive medicine, will together comprise one WTE in heath care and another WTE in 'other activities'.

The results of the survey would have been:

$$(.20\ HC + .80\ OA) + (.80\ HC + .20\ OA) = (1 \times HC) + (1 \times OA)$$

where HC = health care

OA = "other activities".

In the same situation the pragmatic approach would have yielded:

$$(.50\ OA + .50\ HC) + (.50\ HC + .50\ OA) = (1 \times HC) + (1 \times OA).$$

Table 4 illustrates changes over recent years in the types of activities carried out by medical professionals.

An even more detailed breakdown of activities is possible. For example, health care can be divided into outpatient care (in private practices or in polyclinics not administered by a hospital) and in-hospital treatment. At the beginning of 1985, for example, the first category of activities (outpatient care) represented 64% of all health care (14 783 of 23 242 WTE in health care). From Table 4 it is clear that only about 76% of all medical graduates

Table 4. Activities of medical practitioners at beginning of year

	1975 Absolute number	Index 1975 = 100	% of the total	1985 Absolute number	Index 1975 = 100	% of the total	1979 Absolute number	Index 1975 = 100	% of the total	1982 Absolute number	Index 1975 = 100	% of the total
Type of activity												
1. Health care	15 566	100	83	23 242	149	76	18 796	121	81	21 338	137	79
2. Other activities	2 139	100	11	3 759	176	12	2 950	138	13	3 062	143	11
3. "Non-active"	1 085	100	6	3 745	345	12	1 442	133	6	2 521	233	9
Total	18 790	100		30 746	114		23 188	123		26 921	143	

Source: Cathologic University of Louvain, Research Unit "Socio-économie de la Santé.

are working directly with patients to provide health care, and that this proportion is decreasing.

Consequently, the latter figure is a much more accurate basis for calculating the number of inhabitants per doctor. In 1985, for example, this ratio would have exceeded 420 (rather than being around 320 according to the standard indicator, i.e. the total number of doctors). The former ratio is much less disquieting than the traditional indicator plainly based on all doctors. This is an important difference when international comparisons are being made, given that some countries draw a clear distinction between public health activities and private practice.

1.2.4 Qualifications

With the traditional approach, it would be appropriate to refer to specialization. However, the term is becoming inadequate since, in addition to specialists, there are trainee-specialists doing work more closely resembling that of their future colleagues than that of GPs. It is therefore wrong to group them together with the latter. Moreover, a distinction is now made between ordinary GPs and those who are 'retrained' or 'approved' and who enjoy a status similar to that of specialists, particularly with regard to the medical insurance system. Moreover, simply classifying medical practitioners on the basis of their qualifications does not take adequate account of the proportion of them actually available to patients. In order to obtain a clearer view of the actual situation, the classification must be based not only on qualifications but also on the *type of activity* – as is done in Table 5. From this table it can be seen that the proportion of general practitioners is growing at the expense of specialists, but that it is still below the 50% level of all graduates including trainee-specialists, namely, for those involved in health care (and thus available to help patients). This trend is due to a slightly faster increase in the number of general practitioners working elsewhere than in health care and to falling activitiy rates. Turning to the certification granted to 'retrained' general practitioners after an initial refresher course, 450–650 such applications are approved each year. At the end of 1982, 47% of the general practitioners were 'approved'.

Bearing in mind that this certification has involved only younger doctors over the past 5 years, it is apparent that some 70% of graduates who do not go on to specialize undertake this additional qualification in general medicine, a qualification that allows them to charge higher fees.

The seemingly very significant increase shown in Table 5 in the number of trainee-specialists may be only a temporary phenomenon, since the authorities are now tending to reduce the number of available positions rather than increase them (see Chap. 2).

1.3 Geographical Distribution

The geographical distribution of medical manpower may be analysed either in terms of the degree of urbanization or on a regional basis.

Table 5. Qualifications and activities of medical practioners 1975–1982 (beginning of the year) expressed as WTE[a]. For each category of medical practitioner there are three columns of figures: an absolute figure, percentage of the total number of doctors with the same qualifation, and percentage of the total number of doctors carrying out the same activity. Columns 10, 11 and 12 give totals in absolute figures, percentage of the total, and a total for each activity

Year and type of activity	Qualifications General practitioners			Specialists			Trainee-specialists			Total (including doctors practising dentistry)		
	1	2	3	4	5	6	7	8	9	10	11	12
1975												
1. Health care activities	6 169	76.8	39.6	7 289	88.0	46.8	1 885	100	12.1	15.566	84.5	100
2. Other activities	1 457	18.1	68.12	671	8.1	31.4	–	–	–	2 139	11.6	100
3. Non-active	412	5.1	56.1	323	3.9	43.9	–	–	–	723	4.0	100
Total[b]	8.031	100	43.6	8 279	100	44.9	1 885	100	10.2	18 429[b]	100	100
1985												
1. Health care activities	10 336	68.6	44.5	10 021	78.8	43.1	2 697	100	11.6	23 242[c]	75.6	100
2. Other activites	2 622	17.4	69.8	1 131	8.9	30.1	–	–	–	3 759	12.2	100
3. Non-active[c]	2 116	14.0	56.5	1 566	12.3	41.8	–	–	–	3 745	12.2	100
Total[d]	15 074	100	49.0	12 718	100	41.4	2 697	100	8.8	30 746[c,d]	100	100

a Source: Research Unit "Socio-économie de la Santé" of the Catholic University Louvain.
b Including 234 doctors practising dentistry, not including graduates aged over 75 years (estimated at approximately 350).
c Including 257 doctors practising dentistry.
d Including graduates more than 75 years of age (947 in all).

1.3.1 Distribution with Urbanization as the Criterion

It is a well-known fact that higher levels of urbanization, reflected in densely populated municipalities, are associated with a greater density of specialists, whereas GPs are almost uniformly distributed on a graph ranking municipalities in order of size. This is shown clearly by Fig. 1, which plots the information from Table 6. At the upper end of the urbanization scale, specialists are twenty times more densely distributed than they are in the smallest municipalities, where general practioners are in the majority. In 1976, it was only in municipalities of 30 000 or more people that specialists began to dominate, eventually outnumbering general practitioners three to one in the category covering the eight municipalities with 100 000 or more inhabitants. In that year, more than half of all specialiasts were practising in municipalities of more than 70 000 people, home to approximately a quarter of the population. More than 80% were to be found in municipalities of more than 25 000 inhabitants – where half the country's population lives.

1.3.2 Regional Distribution

1.3.2.1 The Choice of Indicators

In analyses of regional distribution, the size and geographical location of the administrative units sampled influence both the results of the statistics and the conclusions drawn from them. Very large units will mean a smoothing out of differences, although those that do remain are often significant enough to form the basis of specific health or budgetary policies.

Examination of units lower in the administrative hierarchy, e.g. 'provinces' or arrondissements yields more detailed information, but it is then difficult to obtain an overall picture. Nor are such units a suitable basis for policy-making, since they do not determine the size of their own budgets. Nevertheless, they have formed the basis of a medical cadastre that, as it has become more detailed, has become of increasing interest to graduates looking for a suitable place to set up practice. Indeed, the market is saturated to such an extent that young doctors now have to analyse the situation in smaller and smaller units, right down to individual municipalities or even to specific areas within them.

Any analysis of geographical distribution that groups all doctors together will be misleading. Indeed, the population–doctor' ratio is too often regarded as an indicator of 'average number of potential patients', which gives a completely false picture of the market and of the extent of competition. This ratio, and its mirror image, the 'doctor–population ratio', should in fact be calculated separately for general practitioners and specialists. Moreover, if they are to be used as guidelines or to advise on the possibilities of setting up practice, they should cover only those doctors actually treating patients. Such a restriction can considerably alter the statistics, and thus their interpretation in terms of the potential for establishing a practice.

1.3.2.2 Some Statistics on Belgium

There are three major linguistic, cultural, economic and social regions in Belgium. Medical coverage is lower in Flanders, particularly for historical reasons, and very extensive in

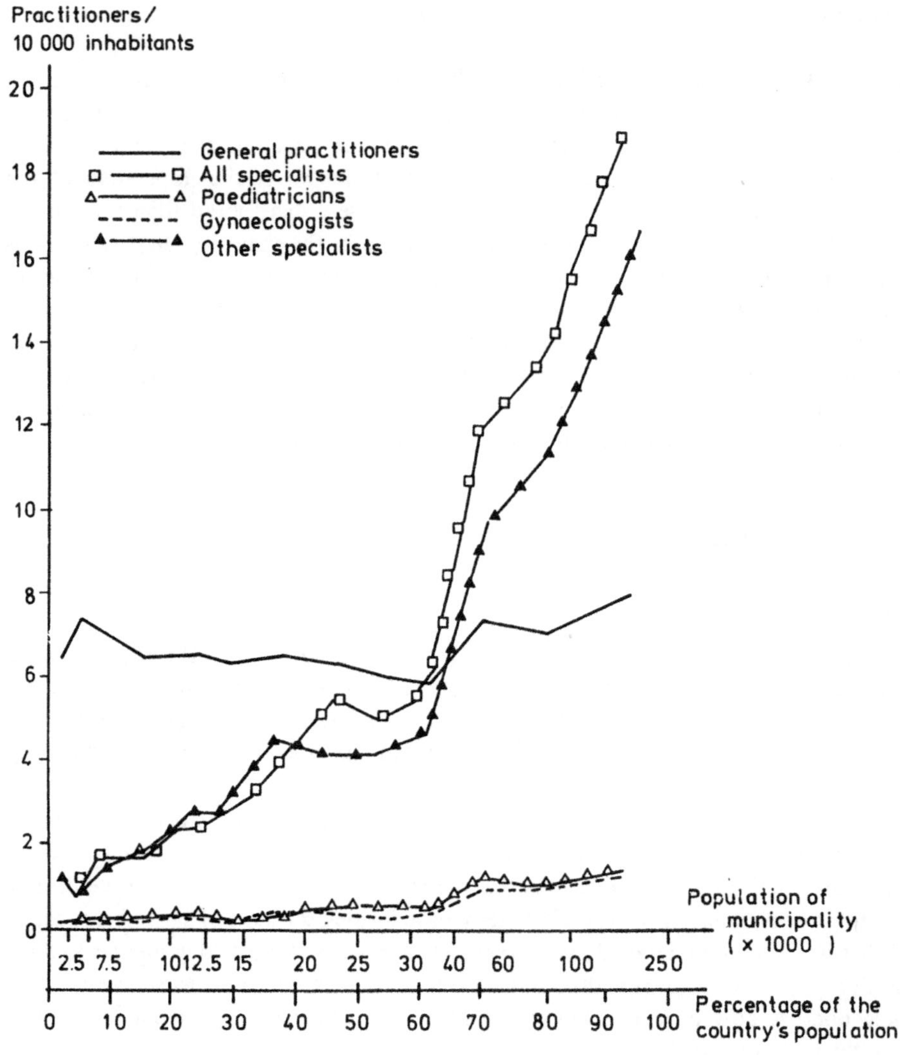

Fig. 1

Brussels, the capital, an administrative agglomeration separated from its hinderland, and the site of three medical schools. There is an even more striking difference in the case of specialists, particularly between Brussels and the rest of the country (three times as many per capita, but also between Wallonia and Flanders (44% more in the former).

Table 7 bears out the point made in Sect. 1.3.2.1, showing how regional differences in the number of doctors in a given area vary depending on whether coverage includes all graduates or only those physicians actually treating patients. It is apparent from the table that the specialists in Brussels are the only group virtually unaffected by the change in statistical parameter; in all other groups, restricting coverage to those doctors actually treating patients yields an 'average number of potential patients' 24%–80% higher than that calculated on the basis of the total number of physicians. The difference is particularly

Table 6. Geographical distribution by size of municipality, size of population, and amount of medical manpower in 1974 and 1976

Size of municipality (1976)	Cumulative percentages Population 1974 and 1976	General practitioners 1974	General practitioners 1976	Specialists 1974	Specialists 1976
⩽ 7 500 inhabitants	10	10.2	10.5	1.6	1.8
⩽ 12 000 inhabitants	25	23.8	24.7	5.3	5.9
⩽ 25 000 inhabitants	50	47.2	48.7	18.1	19.4
⩽ 70 000 inhabitants	75	71.5	72.2	43.2	44.1
	Upper quartile				
> 70 000 inhabitants	25	28.5	27.8	56.8	55.9

Source: X. Le Roy, *L'accès aux soins médicaux*, vol. II, p 22.

Table 7. Number of inhabitants per doctor by region and activity – 1982

Region	General practitioners	*Index*[a]	Specialists	*Index*[a]	Degree of specialization[b]
1. *All doctors with a given qualification* (end 1982)					
Flanders	885	*175*	1 208	*293*	.42
Wallonia	691	*137*	848	*206*	.45
Brussels	505	*100*	411	*100*	.55
Belgium	758		914		.45
2. *Doctors treating patients* (Jan. 1, 1982)					
Flanders	1 274	*140*	1 567	*372*	.45
Wallonia	990	*109*	1 049	*249*	.49
Brussels	911	*100*	421	*100*	.68
Belgium	1 123		1 091		.50

[a] Relative to Brussels = 100.
[b] Not including trainee-specialist.
Sources: 1. Cabinet du Ministre des Affaires sociales, *Analyse de l'offre médicale de médecins, pharmaciens, dentistes et kinésithérapeutes,* 1983, p. 22; 2. Leroy, X., *Densités et activitiés des médecins en Belgique, Situation actuelle,* Paris, December 1983, Cahier de sociologie et de démographie médicales.

marked in the case of general practitioners in Brussels, who are often incorrectly assumed to be treating patients when in fact they are engaged in research, in-service training, preventive medicine and administrative tasks within various government bodies.

At the level of individual arrondissements, i.e. administrative units with populations ranging from 50 000 to over a million, the change of statistical parameter means only a slightly greater spread between the extreme values for avarage numbers of potential patients as far as GPs are concerned (a ratio of 1 : 1.8) but a much greater variation in the case of specialists. Here, the ratio rises to 1 : 20 if Brussels is included and is 1 : 12 if the capital is excluded.

1.4 Future Prospects

Future trends are forecast in three stages:

1. The number of graduates in the future
2. The career choices of these graduates, broken down by qualification (at least separate statistics for GPs and specialists, or with more detailed breakdowns into the various specialities)
3. Availability of physicians covering age and sex structure, the corresponding mortality and the professional activities that will be carried out by the survivors

1.4.1 Forecast of the Number of Future Graduates

The calculations distinguish between (a) Belgians and foreigners and (b) the French- and Dutch-speaking graduates. In each case three forecasts have been made, based on the success rates of medicine and, from 1992, on an even number of graduates until 2000 (scenario C) or a drop of 10%–20% of that number (scenarios B and A). A total of 6250 new doctors will graduate, i.e. will be authorized to practise in Belgium (irrespective of whether or not they are foreigners), over the 5 years from 1986 to 1990. There will be fewer graduates each year, the number dropping from approximately 1500 in 1983 to something over 1000 in 1990.

1.4.2 Forecast of Career Choice of the Newly Qualified

Given the increasingly severe approval criteria for training institutes and training schedules (see Chap. 2), the number of trainee-specialists is unlikely to increase in the future, so that the maximum number of new specialists will remain static; in 1986 the law decreed a rate of 40% of specialists. If this rate is strictly maintained, the number of posts would drop due to the decreasing number of graduates; however, the rate might also be considered a minimum threshold. The computations are based on 40% entering speciality practice; if the rule is not enforced as a ceiling rate, then new forecasts should be made.

1.4.3 Forecast of the Number of Doctors up Until 2000

Given the trend to lower activity rates and the extent to which physicians currently perform activities other than patient care, we felt it essential to provide two separate forecasts of the number of doctors:

Table 8. Forecasted breakdown of new medical graduates by nationality and carrer choice (with full medical degrees)

Year of graduation	Belgians and foreigners A	C
1985–1989	6 136	6 361
1990–1994	4 585	5 226
1995–1999	4 180	5 225
2000–2004	4 180	5 225

A: Before 1992, low success rates; after 1992, stabilisation of forecasted graduates minus 20%.
C: Before 1992, high success rates; after 1992, stabilisation of forecasted graduates.

1. The total number, irrespective of the activities they carry out
2. The number of doctors actually working, particularly those involved only in patient care (in WTE)

Information concerning the assuptions on which these detailed forecasts were made and the methods used to calculate them may be requested from our study unit.

These forecasts are summarized in Table 9, which shows the significant difference between the total number of graduates and those actually active, particularly in the field of health care. Indeed, if there is a continued decrease in the activity rate, only 86% of the available physicians will actually be working (as against 92% 10 years earlier).

2 Supply Management Policies

In Belgium, no regulations have yet been introduced with the aim of directly controlling the increased manpower supply, and the classical approaches in this field have not been resorted to. Access to medical school, the right to practise, and the choice of area in which to do so all remain open to the individual, hampered only in some cases by such specific factors as significant academic failure during training the the difficulty of finding work.

There are, however, certain regulations that indirectly limit access to the profession: the length of a degree course and restrictions on specialization.

Finally, use has been made of an approach that, while quite efficient, in no way restricts individual freedom, i.e. the provision of information, both on the choice of degree course and on the choice of location for doctors' practices.

Table 9. Forecasts of the number of doctors under 75 years old by qualification and type of activity

Category of doctors	Actual situation (1985)	Forecasts in thousands (1990)	(2000)
1. *Total (all doctors)*[a]	29 800	34.5	39.0–40.9
2. *Non-active*			
– Based on 19.85%	2 800	3.5	4.5
– Based on increasing percentages (linear regressions)		5.2	11.1–11.4
3. *Active*	27 000	30.1–30.3	31.8–33.5
4. *General practitioners*			
– Total	14 645	17.8	21.3–22.5
– Those practising health care	10 336	12.5	14.7–15.5
5. *Specialists*			
– Total	12 226	13.9	15.3–16.3
– Those active in health care (including out-patient and hospital work)	10 021	11.3	12.8–13.2
6. *Trainee-specialists*	2 697		

[a] Including doctors practising dentistry.

2.1 Absence of Compulsion

2.1.1 Entry to Courses

With the aim of making university study more generally available, a large number of measures have been taken to make it easier to study. Although there is not selection whatever at this initial stage, selection does nevertheless occur later on.

2.1.1.1 The Sacred Cow of General Access to Universities

There has been a systematic effort to make university education available to all – to the point where it has become a kind of political football. Examples include:

1. The lowering of financial barriers: University fees as such are only Bfrs 17 000 annually, and while the student's family does have to pay such additional costs as board and lodging, books, and course equipment, a small number of scholarships do exist to provide poorer students with financial aid.
2. The elimination of geographical distance as a barrier: Belgium probably leads the world in the number of medical schools for its population – seven full schools for 10 million

inhabitants. Moreover, there has been a "hiving off' of courses to make access to them even easier for the population: there are a total of 11 cities where students can begin to study medicine.

3. The abolition of examination-based barriers: In order to limit the impact of too early a concentration on less strenous subjects, an approach more frequently adopted by poorer students, secondary education has been reformed to provide greater equality of opportunity to all students and to allow access to university to all those succeeding in secondary eduction.

We are not concerned here with the success or failure of this democratization policy. Whatever effect it may have had on improving access to, and success at university for students from poorer families, there has been an undeniably impressive growth in the number of university students: the number of Belgian students jumped from 22 000 in 1955 to 80 000 in 1980, i.e. multiplying by a factor of 3.7 in a quarter of a century. This trend engendered corresponding growth in the number of medical students, albeit less rapid, the multiplication factor being only 2.6 over the same period (calculated on the basis of doctorate years).

Moreover, access to university has become a symbol of individual freedom and a kind of social triumph that no political party has been prepared to tamper with. In spite of the favourable light in which the "numerus clausus" idea (i.e. limitation of admission to a university on the basis of grades) is viewed by professional organizations and – intellectually – by a number of policital and academic figures, there has never been a serious attempt to draft the appropriate legislation.

An additional factor is that certain political groups have deliberately chosen to allow the medical profession to become overpopulated – with the evident aim of thus destroying one of the bastions of the traditionally wealthy bourgeois elite. This desire, however, has never appeared in black and white.

2.1.1.2 Natural Selection Nevertheless Takes Place

Access to university may be relatively easy but it does not, for all that, guarantee success. Natural selection, in terms of the effort expended and the ability to learn, comes into its own. Instead of acting prior to admission to university, its effects can be seen throughout the course of study, particularly during the first 2 or 3 years.

In consequence, no valid international comparisons can be made of the number of people entering for the first preliminary examination – since the expected success rate in individual countries gives the number of students a completely different significance. Whereas almost 95% of French students entering the first preliminary examination go on to graduate, this rate is only approximately 45% in Belgium. It used to be even lower: approximately 38% of classes in the late 1970s (the rate being calculated on the basis of blocks of students not necessarily coming from the same entering class).

Moreover, there are changes over time in these rates. For example, the success rate for Dutch-speaking Belgian students climbed from 38% to 52% in 10 years, whereas it remained stable, at about 39%, for French-speaking students. This trend is a result of various changes during the course of studies. The fluctuations are not linked to those in the absolute number of students beginning the study of medicine: a decrease in the number of students does not necesarily improve the success rate.

2.1.2 Admission to the Medical Profession

Restrictions on entry to the profession can cover the following three fields: approval to provide health care, approval to treat patients under a sickness insurance scheme, and the opportunity to specialize.

2.1.2.1 Approval to Provide Health Care

Although certain formalities must be completed before graduates can treat patients (official endorsement of their diploma and registration in the roll of physicians), these are usually mere formalities, and there is therefore an almost automatic right to practise. Until the end of the 1970s, this freedom amounted in effect to a guarantee of work and thus of income. This is no longer entirely the case, given the difficulty of finding a job or a place to practice (see Sect. 2.1.3).

2.1.2.2 Patient Care Under a Sickness Insurance Scheme

Patients may seek treatment from whatever doctor they choose, while still having the majority of the medical bills paid by the sickness insurance scheme. This is true of the national schemes covering the majority of workers: employees, public servants, and the self-employed, together with their families. A few schmes stipulate that treatment be carried out by certain approved physicians. These include the railways and armed forces schemes.

In other words, any doctor can make out a bill, and the official fee will automatically be reimbursed to the patient by the sickness insurance scheme (except for the patient's share). Moreover, patients may consult specialists directly, without being referred by their family doctor and without any change in the conditions of reimbursement.

Although agreements ('conventions') are negotiated periodically, this process involves only an undertaking by physicians to respect the scale of fees negotiated between their representatives and the sickness insurance schemes. Moreover, this undertaking is automatic for all those who do not expressly state their refusal to be bound by these fee scales. Once a quorum of participating physicians has been reached, these fee scales become applicable to all doctors in the region concerned.

Until a new convention has been negotiated, and its provisions can come into force, patients continue to receive medical bills that are reimbursed in accordance with the previously negotiated fee scale. In a number of cases the practitioners' trade unions have advocated to raise fees above the official tariff; usually, however, some agreement is reached.

2.1.2.3 Opportunity to Provide Specialized Treatment

Although all medical graduated are legally entitled to provide any kind of medical care, such specialized treatment is reimbursed by the sickness insurance scheme only where it has been provided by approved specialists working within their own field of specialization. It is therefore essential that a doctors specialize if the wishes to provide a certain type of treatment. Accordingly, the increasing difficulty encountered in specializing becomes a definite obstacle preventing a number of graduates from practising in the field of their choice (see Sect. 2.2).

2.1.3 Limitations on Setting up Practice and on Finding Work

2.1.3.1 No Legal Restrictions

There are no regulations to prevent a doctor from establishing his own practice or taking a job in a hospital. In theory, the doctor's freedom is completely untrammelled in this respect. A draft 'Medical Practice Law' permitting doctors to set up practice only if licensed to do so on the basis of the 'needs of the population', was suggested by professional bodies in the late 1970s. Official approval was not forthcoming and the proposal was therefore dropped.

Quite a few arguments can be advanced against any policy seeking to limit supply by imposing authoritarian restrictions on the establishment of private practices; they will be listed in Sect. 3.4.2.1.

2.1.3.2 Actual Obstacles

Even in the absence of legal restrictions, it is not easy to find work as a doctor because of the growing saturation of the market. It is becoming more and more difficult to find a suitable place to set up a practice as every region already has more than enough doctors. Graduates therefore have to find individual areas where a relatively lower degree of saturation exists (see Sect. 2.3). This is more easily done in Flanders than in Wallonia or in Brussels.

In the case of access to hospital posts, this is again a field without legal standards dictating a specific ratio of graduates, or WTEs, to beds. This omission is surely a surprising one at a time when other hospital functions are very strictly controlled by standards covering staff levels relative to the number of beds. In the absence of compulsory standards, the young graduate therefore depends on the goodwill of hospital decision-makers and on any increase that may occur in the number of hospitals. In either care, the young doctor's changes are poor.

As far as obtaining work in an existing hospital is concerned, there is nothing to prevent senior doctors already employed by the hospital from running an understaffed department with too many patients rather than sharing work and income with young colleagues. We have also been made aware of cases where posts have been reserved for future colleagues still at medical school, thanks to their family connections or because they come from the immediate area. It would therefore be in the interest of not only public health but also social justice for young doctors were standards to be introduced governing the ratio of medical personnel to the number of beds, the specialities of such doctors, their obligation to be on call, etc.

As for any increase in the number of hospitals, this cannot be counted on to supply additional employment. Indeed, there are no prospects of expansion whatever, for the following reasons:

1. The standards used as the basis for hospital planning have already been greatly exceeded: over the whole country, surplus capacity amounts to 20%.
2. Given the budget deficit, the government has decided on a series of measures designed to prevent new budget overruns. The opening of new hospitals already planned and under construction (involving 15.4% additional overcapacity) is therefore now in jeop-

ardy. These wards will be given permission to open only if they are replacing other hospital beds so as not to exceed the number of approved beds as of 1 July 1982. Operating costs will not be underwritten by the government if beds are brought into service without permission and without proof that other beds have been taken out of service or converted to other use.

3. The use of existing beds has further been limited by a compulsory reduction in the number of days spent in hospital that can be reimbursed by the sickness insurance schemes: a 3% reduction 1983 and a 5% reduction in 1984 (4% and 6% respectively in the psychiatric sector). There is also a limit on transfers to those departments usually underoccupied. Hospitals may combine to achieve reductions, for example, by closing individual departments.
4. In order to encourage a drop in hospital capacity, compensation is available for the closure of hospitals or health-care units, for not commissioning hospitals or units now under construction, or for the abandonment of projects already planned.
5. In addition to the reductions in capacity imposed in 1983 and 1984 (see point 3 above), there are a number of incentives to encourage further reduction in hospital beds by allowing and aiding the conversion of hospitals into nursing homes. Payments for nursing care can be made to approved old people's homes (or to integrated services for home health care) as a means of shortening, or avoiding entirely, any stays in hospital. An agreement to cover treatment costs can now replace charges calculated on the basis of hospital days for those hospitalized patients whose condition no longer requires hospital care. A Royal Decree made it possible to establish on a departmental basis the criteria, in terms of duration of hospitalization, governing changes from one such agreement to another. Provisional approval for new nursing-home beds could be given only where these were matched by an 'equivalent' reduction in the number of hospital beds. It was later decided that the closing of one hospital bed would be sufficient grounds for approving two new nursing-home beds.

2.2 Indirect Restrictive Regulations

Two measures, taken ostensibly to improve the quality of medical training, will in effect make medical courses less attractive and so encourage fewer students to take them. These concern the length of courses and restrictions on specialization. Moreoever, measures to limit output and expenditure on health will help to make the profession less financially attractive.

2.2.1 The Length of Courses: New Obstacles

Medical courses were already lengthy: a basic 7 years, not counting any necessary repeated subjects or the additional years required for any specialization. While there has been no official change in the length of course, a ministerial decree in late 1982 established new criteria for GPs wishing to obtain special qualifications enabling them to administer certain forms of general medical treatment (and thus to charge higher fees) to patients who were members of sickness insurance schemes. The decree requires specific training in the following fields: human and social aspects of general medical practice, pathology and the appropriate basic therapy for given age-groups, long-term therapy for the chronically ill, emergency medical treatment, epidemiology, preventive medicine and prophylactic treatment, medical legislation, and the organization of a general practice. The decree also laid down a 2-year period of 'supervised medical practice'.

Although the decree does not state that this specific training must follow the basic course, or that supervised medical practice is incompatible with running one's own practice, medical students see these provisions as constituting a 2-year delay before they can exercise their profession in complete independence. Moreover, fears have been voiced that indirect restrictions will be encountered in the form of a shortage of physicians who are prepared to act as mentors to young doctors beginning their 'supervised' career. This fear is enhanced by the existence of a draft European Directive calling for a minimum of 2 years' additional training in general medicine, following the 6 years of basic training required under the 1975 directive.

2.2.2 Access to Specialization: An Additional Hurdle in the Offing

Officially, there is no limit to the number of students in training courses, but in practice there are already a number of ways in which these are limited, and further restrictions are being prepared. The potential for specialization is, in fact, restricted by the avaiability of suitable training institutes for young doctors.

There are three levels at which regulations constitute obstacles:

1. *Applicants* are required to submit their proposed training schedule to the appropriate committee in the Ministry of Public Health. On completion of the training course they must also apply for licensing, either as a specialist or as an approved GP, in particular enclosing statements by the training supervisor(s). The committee then examines the applicant's entire file.
2. The *training supervisors* must be approved by the Ministry of Public Health after obtaining the opinion of a board within the Ministry which assesses these specialists on the basis of their qualifications, functions and publications, as well as their participation in scientific associations and congresses.
3. The *training department* must also be approved, following the same procedure. General criteria with respect to these various approval formalities were also set out in decrees, while a whole series of decrees have established specific criteria for each speciality. These criteria stipulate the minimum size of departments and of their practice lists, the maximum number of trainee-specialists per training supervisor and per health-care unit, the existence of certain techniques or types of health care, and the obligation to keep registers and medical files for each patient and for each diagnosis.

These regulations themselves have already limited available posts. The board is attempting to restrict *future* admissions by defining 'need' on the basis of criteria that have yet to be published.

2.2.3 Restricting "Output" of Services

Faced with an explosive increase in government health expenditure – particularly difficult to bear in a period of economic crisis – successive governments have applied a number of financial 'tourniquets' concerning health-care financing, prices, the level of consumption, supply, output and income. A number of measures will make the profession less attractive and could eventually discourage those who want to enter it more for the financial than for the spiritual rewards that it brings. However, since this report's terms of reference do not include a detailed analysis of techniques for limiting health-care expenditure, we will only mention the various measures.

2.2.3.1 Financing Health Care

A number of discussions were held in early 1984 to examine ways of financing hospital care. Several systems have already been examined, but the relevant reports have yet to be published.

2.2.3.2 Prices

Negotiations between doctors and sickness insurance schemes have often resulted in 'moderate' increases – in line, incidentally, with requests for moderation addressed to other professional categories. Lower fees have been agreeed on in those sectors with very clear increases in output, such as clinical biology.

2.2.3.3 Consumption Levels

A range of measures have been taken to make the patient pay more for health care. There is now a more widespread requirement to pay part of the cost, involving a lowering of the income ceiling (in the case of widows, retired persons and invalids) for cheaper medical treatment; an increase in the patient's own contribution for certain types of health care (general medicine, physiotherapy, hospitalization, etc.); and pressure put on doctors to collect this patient contribution.

2.2.3.4 Limitation of Supply

Clinical-biology and nuclear-medicine laboratories must now be approved, and there are quality controls on the work of clinical biologists. The planning and limitations of hospital beds has been covered in Sect. 2.1.3.

2.2.3.5 Limitations on Output

A limit on the number of analyses that can be requested simultaneously has been introduced, as have been checks on output in the form of 'medical profiles' (to detect 'hyper-producers' and, at a later stage, 'hyper-prescribers' and 'hyper-consumers').

2.2.3.6 Limitations on Income

Steps have been taken to discourage tax evasion; e.g. a requirement to keep records of fees collected.

2.3 Information

A novel approach has been adopted in Belgium to slow down the exaggerated growth in the supply of doctors and to permit better use of the medical manpower available. Information is provided in such a way as to obtain the desired results without infringing on either individual freedom of choice or the adaptive flexibility of market mechanisms, yet without resorting to restrictive regulations. An additional advantage of this technique is that it permits rapid adaptation to market changes. It is therefore obviously a much more flexible approach than one in which laboriously draw-up regulations have to be modified. This information can help individuals make the necessary decisions at three crucial points in their career: the choice of university course, the choice of a speciality, and the choice of an area in which to set up practice.

2.3.1 Pre-university Information

2.3.1.1 Content

Young people who are deciding which university course to take cannot be allowed to chase rainbows. The information traditionally supplied on the length of courses must therefore be supplemented by additional information on the prospects of employment and income after graduation. This information can be based on the current situation but, ideally, it should also analyse future trends and provide a forecast of market conditions, in spite of the risk involved in making such predictions; i.e. it should be possible to provide forecasts of medical manpower, consumption and output for 7–10 years ahead.

2.3.1.2 Information Flow

Since 1973, a number of studies have drawn attention to the dangers associated with the growing number of medical students and have made the relevant authorities aware of the problem. In order to bring market forces into play, there is a need for wide dissemination of the results of such studies, and the Ministry of Social Affairs has twice undertaken extensive publicity campaigns.

The universities, during their open days for secondary-school pupils, have been a traditional channel for providing young people with information. It would therefore be wise to encourage cooperation with the universities. This would require a fundamental change in the way they are financed; rather than a subsidy based on the number of students, they should receive an overall lump sum to cover their actual costs.

2.3.1.3 Effectiveness of This Information Technique

This information technique, which safeguards the principles of free choice and unrestricted access to university study, appears to have achieved considerable success. Since 1977–1978, the number of entrants to the first intermediate examination in medical science has fallen by 45% for French-speaking students and by 25% for Dutch-speaking students.

2.3.2 *Information on Specialization*

Chance factors, such as a training post becoming available, may dictate the choice of speciality, but the choice can also be made easier, and can be influenced, by providing better information on the current situation and future prospects in given specialities. This information includes the age structure of practitioners, the specialist: population ratio and estimates of how this will evolve, predicted trends in legislation affecting doctors' work or income, and the ease of access to hospital beds. Some work along these lines has already been done.

2.3.3 *Information on Setting up Practice*

The decision on where to practice can be a key one for a successul careeer and now, at a time of growing saturation, it requires considerably more care and thought than it used to. In addition to the personal characteristics of graduates and their preference for working with a given type of patient, a helpful factor in decision-making can be a thorough understanding of specific aspects of the health system. It is therefore vital to establish very detailed registers covering the health system, to analyse them on a regional basis and to make them available for consultation to the new generation of doctors through a decentralized system of information offices.[2]. This is described in Sect. 3.4.2.2.

3 Models Relevant to the Health System

There are subtle relationships between supply, consumption and various socioeconomic variables (Sect. 3.1). If such relationships can be determined, they may provide a useful basis for manpower policies (Sect. 3.4). However, such relationships can hardly be expected to result in a clear model of 'needs', since this is an ambiguous concept which varies over time; in particular, it is dependent on the extent to which the health system has evolved (Sect. 3.2).

It is therefore adviseable to work out a number of future scenarios regarding the way in which the components of the health system are likely to evolve (Sect. 3.3), and to draw conclusions from these regarding the policie to be promoted (Sect. 3.4).

3.1 *Relationship Between Supply, Demand and Environment*

General studies of the medical profession as a whole have shown the effect of factors external to the health system on the geographical distribution of doctors in the various regions, but they were carried out some time ago and are too general in scope.

---

2 Such a system operated throughout Belgian universities for a few months and is now available through the University of Louvain, which makes the information available to all universities.

Separate, more detailed studies have subsequently been made of general medicine and specialized medicine. In practice, these two factors of the health system do not follow the same development, and they should therefore be treated separately when the consumption of health care and the other characteristics of their environment are examined.

Although they concern more significant groups, the findings relating to the two sectors are deficient in the sense that they come from studies which were not specifically desgined to analyse the distribution of doctors in Belgium. While they enable the supply of doctors to be linked to a number of factors characterizing the consumption of health care or to certain socioeconomic characteristics of the region concerned, the studies were designed for other purposes, and they neglect factors which are known to affect the distribution of doctors, such as the presence nearby of a medical school or of a teaching hospital attached to a university. It is therefore impossible to devise a model which explains or forecasts distribution; we can only tentatively suggest some possible interpretations of the links observed.

3.1.1 The Medical Profession as a Whole

It is not really advisable to include general practitioners and specialist in one analysis in view of the different way in which they are distributed (see above). However, we would like to mention a tentative model that was proposed for this area many years ago, because it related separately to five of the Common Market countries and simultaneously to all the EEC regions. The similarity of the results obtained is striking.

In the study, a stepwise multiple regression analysis was carried out, which involved 17 variables as possible explanatory factors for the ratios of doctors and dentists to the number of inhabitants, and there are certain findings which are common to the various analyses:

- The predominance of cultural factors such as the ratios of university graduates (other than doctors and dentists) or students to the general population and the presence of a medical school
- The proportion of women in the population was related to the density of doctors probably as an index of urbanization
- Urbanization (the proportion of the population living in municipalities with over 20 000 inhabitants) also has an effect as do, in a negative sense, certain indices of ruralism (the proportion of the working population engaged in agriculture and fishing or the proportion of the population living in municipalities with fewer than 5000 inhabitants).
- Purely economic factors such as income per head gross domestic product, or income prospects rarely have an effect.
- Certain indicators which might be regarded as 'need' factors, such as the numbers of young children and elderly people and infant mortality, also rarely have an effect.

The links described above should not be regarded as true causal explanations for the distribution of doctors. The latter are not 'attracted' by the presence of other university graduates or by larger numbers of women. There are probably distribution characteristics common to members of the various professions, who congregate more in certain areas for certain shared reasons which are at present beyond our grasp but which may be linked to urbanization and a high level of services per capita (which would be consistent with the presence of a larger number of women), although the variables specifically designed to measure these two factors were not the most prominent.

Later studies relating solely to Belgium have only indicated a very strong correlation between the doctor-population ratios in 1974 and those in 1976 and 1979, regardless of the indicator chosen, which points to a certain stability in distribution patterns over time, at least during the short period in question.

3.1.2 General and Specialized Medicine

The findings for each of these two sectors relate only to Belgium, first to the country as a whole and then to Flanders and Wallonia separately, the latter two regions forming relatively distinct systems separated by different language and cultural traditions. The supply of doctors is examined in relation to the following factors:

- The socioeconomic characteristics of the regions (in 1974)[3]
- Supply characteristics within each sector (1974, 1976, 1979)
- Consumption characteristics in the sector concerned and the degree of technical sophistication of the medicine practised in the region (1974, 1976, 1979)
- Characteristics of output per doctor (1976 and 1979)

As can be seen, the analyses were normally carried out for more than 1 year and their results are mentioned below only of they are confirmed by the various regional and time-series analyses. Only simple correlations have been calculated.

3.1.2.1 General Medicine

Supply of General Practioners and Regional Characteristics

None of the socioeconomic characteristics of the regions is clearly associated with the GP-population ratios. In many cases, the results relating to Wallonia and Flanders are contradictory.

Our initial working hypothesis was that doctors preferred to practise in areas with a high standard of living and that this was particularly true in the past when, in view of the lack of doctors then existing, the doctors' personal preferences might still have been more important than meeting the needs of the population. Our analyses, however, show that such a link exists only in Wallonia, although the doctor-population ratio there is 26% higher than in the north of the country. Perhaps these findings reflect two different stages in the development of the health system:

---

[3] The factors were as follows: population density, proportion of the population living in towns with more than 10 000 inhabitants (urbanization indicator), percentage of self-employed persons among the insured population (index of ruralism), average incomes, standard of living (a complex indicator obtained from a factorial analysis of 13 variables measuring the types of education available and the scale of public and private services), scales of private wealth, life expectancy of males at birth, endogenous infant mortality, exogenous infant mortality.

1. In Wallonia, the suply of GPs is linked to the standard of living, although there is no shortage of supply in any area. It is not clear whether this link really reflects a tendency among GPs to settle in areas for reasons of personal preference or in the hope (which may be self-deluding – see below) that consumption will expand.
2. In Flanders, which has relatively fewer doctors, the presence of GPs is linked more to the rural character of the area concerned and to a long life expectancy than to certain socioeconomic characteristics reflecting a high standard of living.

Supply of General Practitioners and Consumption of Health Care

Contrary to what is generally thought, there is hardly any correlation between the GP-population ratios and the extent to which general practitioners' services are used. Thus, there is no correlation in the regional data for the country as a whole, while the correlation for Flanders ($r < .45$) is low; in Wallonia, such correlations used to exist but had disappeared in the last year analysed (1979). The geographical distribution therefore relates litte, or no longer at all, to the level of demand as perceived by the patient. This also means that supply cannot always create its own damand contrary to what was previously assumed.

As was to be expected, the presence of a large number of GPs does not lead to greater technical sophistication in the type of care provided. Within each region, there is scarcely any correlation between GP-population ratios and the level of specialization of the care sought, special technical examinations, or the 'technical coefficient' (the number of technical examinations per visit/consultation). The consumption of medicines and the use of physiotherapy are related to GP-population rations only in Flanders.

Supply of General Practitioners and Output Characteristics

"Output" refers to the average number of consultations and visits carried out by each doctor. Output correlates negatively with the GP-population ratios, especially when the country is taken as a whole ($r = -.66$ to $-.81$ depending on the year; $P < .001$) and in Wallonia ($r = -.44$ to $-.85$; $P < .005$).

This conclusion confirms that it is not supply which creates its own demand but, rather, that it is medical practice which is induced to adapt to the conditions prevailing in the system. In fact, an examination of changes over time has shown that whereas supply and consumption developed in a very similar way between 1966 and 1974, a clear divergence has occurred since then; supply has been growing at a much faster rate than consumption, with the result that the average output per GP in terms of consultations and visits has steadily dropped. In addition, the supply of GPs has always been closely related to the percentage of doctor/patient sessions represented by house calls ($r = .51$ to $.72$, depending on the region concerned), which once again demonstrates the way in which general practitioners' work changes to take account of changing doctor-population ratios.

3.1.2.2 Specialized Medicine

Supply of Specialists and Regional Characteristics

Specialist-population ratios are linked above all to urbanization and, negatively, to rural conditions. They are also linked positively to average income but not to standard of living (probably because the latter does not depend on the level of urbanization). There is no link with life expectancy or with the two types of infant mortality. These findings apply to both parts of the country but need to be confirmed by more recent data.

Supply of Specialists and Other Supply Characteristics
There is hardly any relationship between the overall GP-population and specialist-population ratios. The ratios of specialists' practices to the number of inhabitants are closely linked to the scale of specialists' work in hospitals.

Supply of Specialists and Consumption of Health Care
Specialist-population ratios are linked to the extent to which specialists' services are used and to the proportion of all doctors' visits and consultations accounted for by specialists. These links are very clear in Belgium as a whole and in Wallonia but less clear in Flanders (owing mainly to its special situation, whereby many districts, especially those around Brussels are near to well-equipped city centres).

The relationship between supply and the 'technical sophistication' of the care provided (i.e. special technical examinations and the 'technical coefficient')[4] are less clear but still highly significant in the country as a whole. There is scarcely any correlation between specialist-population ratios and the other health care consumption characteristics (medicines, physiotherapy or hospitalization rate).

Supply of Specialists and Output
Overall, the growth rates in the supply and consumption of specialized medicine will vary little between 1974 and 1990. Thus, except for slight fluctuations of less than 10%, the output of health care excluding hospital stays will remain very stable. This contrasts with the scope for working in hospital, which, expressed in terms of the number of beds per specialist, decreased by 30% between 1966 and 1981.

However, the results of the regional analysis differ from the observations based on changes over time. Thus, several indices show a negative correlation between supply and output:

- The ratio of specialists' practices to the population, compared with the *non-hospital* output of specialists (in Belgium as a whole and in Wallonia)[1]
- The number of specialists engaged in *hospital* work, compared with the output of hospital work by the specialists concerned (in the country as a whole and in Wallonia)[5]
- The total input of specialists in *hospital and non-hospital* work, compared with the output of hospital work by specialists (only in Belgium as a whole)[1]

It is therefore clear that, as with GPs, the scale of supply determines the way in which specialists work.

However, in contrast to the situation found with GPs, supply and consumption develop in more or less the same way over time; the greater ambiguity of the results of the regional analyses is partly due to the arbitrary nature of the administrative divisions, which rarely

---

4 Technical coefficient = number of technical items per session with the doctor.
5 These relationships are also found in Flanders if each district is weighted with a coefficient corresponding to the proportion of the population living there.

correspond to the 'health areas' that could be identified in terms of the 'radius of attraction' of medical equipment and the 'migration' of patients over district boundaries. Consequently, average output has up to new been little affected by the growth in supply, even though the scope for influencing the behaviour of consumers is not immediate and varies from one region to another. This conclusion, while quite encouraging for the medical profession, gives some cause for concern as regards the control of public expenditure (see Sect. 3.3.2).

3.2 A Manpower Policy Based on Requirements

The question of the level of requirement always recurs in any discussion on manpower policies. Being able to answer this question is frequently presented as the necessary and sufficient precondition for a coherent policy in this area. However, attempts to assess 'needs' or requirements are very rarely made, owing to the ambiguity of the concept and to the constant changes in the criteria for assessing them.

In the following section some of the possible approaches will be mentioned: staffing levels, replacement needs, relative needs and 'overall' needs.

3.2.1 Staffing Levels

In the case of hospitals and other institutions concerned with health (homes, day nurseries, preventive community health services), the number of persons or WTEs required can be assessed. In Belgium, various studies have been made of this problem, particularly in respect of nursing staff. Since the present study is directed mainly towards macroeconomic needs, little space can be devoted to this subject here. However, it is worth pointing out that staffing level guidelines, based on regulations, exist for most hospital professions with the exception of the medical profession.

If such guidelines were introduced, appropriate to the nature and size of the services concerned, they could contribute to the establishment of an overall manpower policy aimed at distributing work among a larger number of people.

3.2.2 Replacement Requirements

While we do not intend to examine the desirability of the present or likely future number of doctors, it is tempting to forecast simple 'replacement requirements', designed to compensate for 'departures'. Even this straightforward aim, however, comes up against the ambiguity of the 'departure' concept and may lead to false conclusions. Thus, apart from deaths of doctors during their working lives, 'departures' may also relate to the following:

- Older generations only: unless estimates are frequently adjusted this criterion is misleading, since the present generation of elderly doctors is very small and will subsequently be replaced by a larger group

– Doctors leaving the profession before the age of 65: the non-active rate is increasing at all ages and for both sexes; it might be unwise to replace these departures because they might represent a self-regulation of the market when the saturation point has been reached; however, after 5 years or so those departures may be considered as having left for ever, so that new needs may require new graduates.
– 'Average departures', calculated so that all existing manpower can be replaced over a period of some 35 years: if this criterion was applied separately to each speciality it would increase supply in the more modern ones, which have seen a huge influx of specialists in the past few years. Here, too, before this criterion is applied generally it would be necessary to decide whether present levels are desirable and whether the rate of increase should continue in future.

3.2.3 Relative Requirements

Without passing judgement on the desirability of present or estimated future levels, it might be useful and convenient to compare one specific situation with that existing in other regions or in neighbouring countries.

Although interregional or international comparisons enable the present level to be set against a scale of development, they cannot be used to assess whether such a degree of

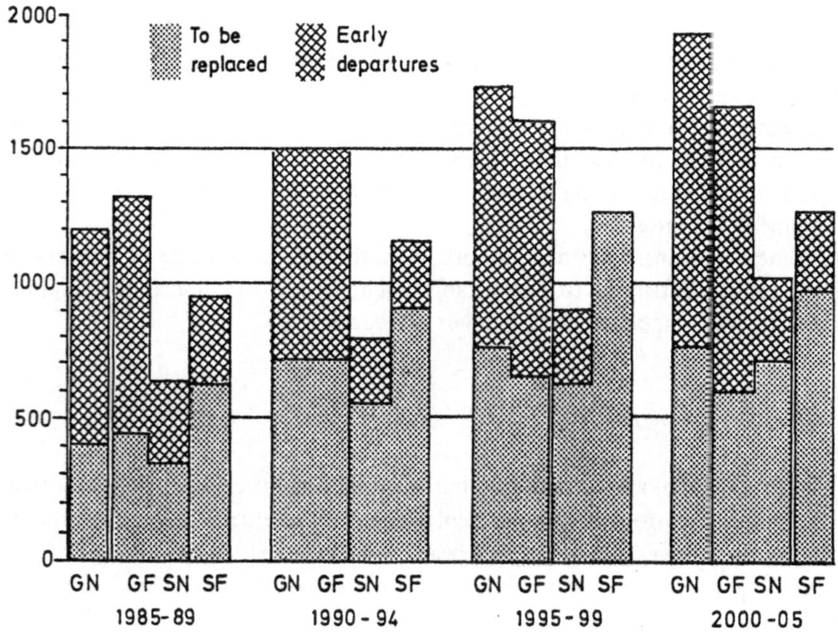

Fig. 2. Departures to be replaced and early departures: high graduate levels. Scenario: Stabilisation of graduate levels after 1992 together with a rising rate of non-activity (regression). Hopefully, the non-active rate will slow down and the true number of early departures will be lower. *G*, general practioners; *S*, specialists; *N*, Dutch-speaking; *F*, French-speaking

development is superior to another or to determine whether it is desirable to 'catch up' with higher doctor-population ratios found elsewhere.

However, at a given time in sociomedical evolution, it might be worthwhile to use this comparative technique in order to arrive at a better geographical distribution of the manpower available. To be of real value, such comparisons must deal not only with simple doctor-population ratios but also with consumption and regional health-care output, two factors which are essential if differences in manpower are to be accurately assessed.

3.2.4 "Overall" Requirements

Essentially, evaluating requirements means forming an opinion as to the desirability of the present or foreseeable future level of manpower. It should be said at the outset that it is illusory to attempt to formulate an abstract standard corresponding to an ideal to be achieved in all circumstances or at all times. The very concept of requirements varies according to whether it is presented and defined by an economist, a member of the profession concerned, or a planner. In common with demographers, they all seek an ideal number of persons or the ideal manpower-population ratio, but each assesses this in the light of his own discipline or his own interests. In each case, the assessment will be based on a set of factors whose criteria and terms of reference change with time, with the stage of development reached, with the acquisition of new knowledge, etc. Thus, the concept is not unambigous and, whatever meaning is selected, the assessment criteria change.

3.2.4.1 Requirements as Seen by the Economist

For an economist, requirements express wishes and levels of possible consumption, according to available resources. The market is organized in such a way as to encourage the expression of such requirements or even to create them and, where possible, to satisfy them. When satisfied, they are replaced by new ones. Requirements are therefore regarded as one of the engines of growth; in the case of medical care, financed to a large extent out of public funds rather than household budgets, they come into conflict with other types of requirements which have to be financed by the community.

In addition, their growth – being more rapid than that of the nation's wealth – places increasing pressure on public finances and, indirectly, on the competitiveness of the undertakings which to a large extent finance them.

3.2.4.2 Requirements as Seen by Members of the Professions

The members of a profession tend to assess a supply situation in the light of the competition which they might face. With this in mind, assessments must be made of operating costs, average incomes and work schedules. By evaluating these criteria it will be possible to determine the working situation of the group analysed, both as regards its development over time and in comparison with other professional groups.

3.2.4.3 Requirements as Seen by the Planner

To determine the number of doctors required at any given time, the planner must employ the following criteria:

- Epidemiological data: the volume of disease requiring health care during a given year, to be treated by the various specialities
- The volume of care required for each of these diagnostic groups, in the light of knowledge available at the time (or of progress likely to be made in that area)
- The productivity of the medical profession.

The requirements determined on this general basis will then be compared with other needs of the country so that a decision can be made, if necessary, regarding the allocation of the limited resources in the economy between competing needs. The planner must therefore take account of the economic constraits. Figure 3 shows how an assessment of overall requirements can be attempted.

3.3 Future Prospects

A rational manpower policy should be based not only on the present situation, so that the supply can be used to the best advantage, but also on that likely to exist in 10 year's time, so that the rules governing access to a profession involving a training period between 7 and 15 years can be suitably adapted. The study of future prospects should include not only manpower but also other aspects of the system such as consumption, needs (if possible) and, perhaps, workloads. The forecasts shown in Table 10, under separate headings for general practitioners and specialists, assume a 40% rate of specilisation for future graduates. The forecasts will have to be adjusted in case of actual rate increase, as might be expected.

3.3.1 Outlook Regarding the Supply of Doctors up to the Year 2000

3.3.1.1 The Situation in 1990

In 1990 there will be over 34 000 medical graduates (one for every 283 inhabitants), of whom some 30 000 will be in usual medical professions, as explained in Sect. 1.4.3. Were the specialisation rate to remain at 40%, these 30 000 will include some 15 000 'GPs' and 13 000 'specialists' and 2000 trainees; these terms have been placed in inverted commas because not all the graduate doctors will be engaged in dispensing health care. If work outside the health-care sector (more common among 'GPs') and the rise in the non-active rate (at every age and among both sexes) are taken into account, the number of doctors dispensing medical care to patients in 1990 will be much lower than the above totals, with 12 450 GPs and 11 300 specialists providing health care, calculated as WTE. This means that the number of GPs will double between 1974 and 1990 the number of specialists will rise by 50%.

3.3.1.2 Outlook for the Year 2000

Any attempt at forecasting for the years following 1990 is very risky, since most of the doctors who will graduate during that decade have not yet started their studies. Any forecasts must therefore be based on assumptions only. Forecasts have been computed following three hypotheses: the number of graduates will remain stable (after 1990 about 1050

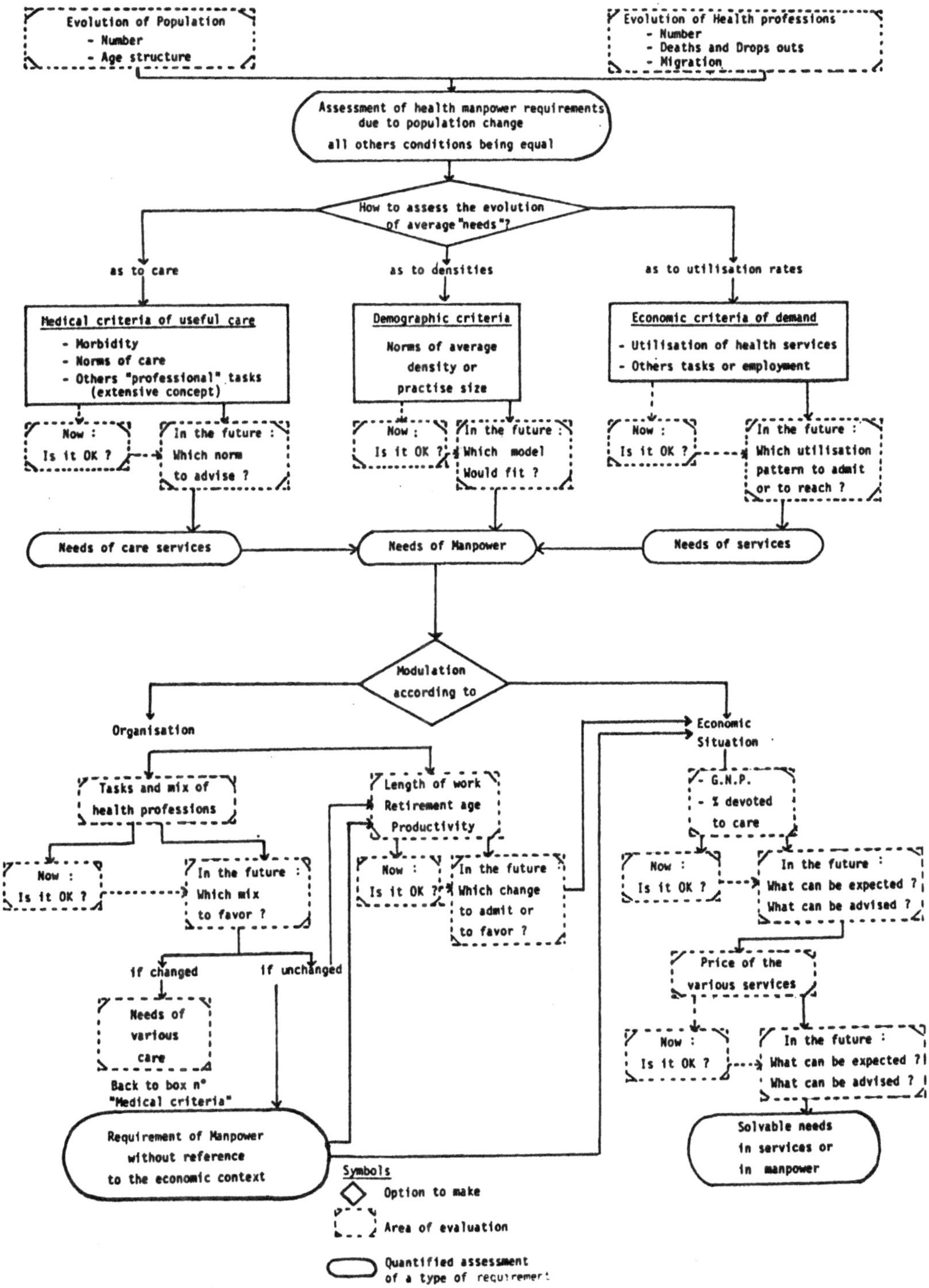

Fig. 3. How to access future requirements of health manpower?

Table 10. Trends and future prospects in general and specialized medicine

General practitioners	1974	1979	1982	1985	1990	2000
Population size (x 10^3)	9772	9848	9856	9858	9740	9623
Supply in WTE (1 Jan)[a]						
– Total (in thousands)[b]	7.8	10.0	12.3	14.9	17.8	21.3
– Active[c]	7.3	9.5	11.1	13.1	14.4	13.7
– Number providing health care[d]	5.7	7.2	8.8	10.2	11.9–11.1	14.0
– Inhabitants/WTE[e]	1660	1337	1094	954	782–836	657
Consumption per inhabitant per year						
Sessions[f]						
– slow growth[f]				5.03	5.11	5.26
– rapid growth[f]	4.74	4.98	4.99	5.14	5.39	5.95
Output per WTE						4762
Sessions per year[h]	7888	6589	5447	5000	4440	4085
Sessions per week	175	146	121	111	99	106
Work schedule: hours per week						
– Total number of hours worked	65					
– of which: dispensing health care	51					
Income from private work[i]						
– millions of BF (1985 prices)	1.97	1.91	1.49	1.38		
Specialists	**1974**	**1979**	**1982**	**1985**	**1990**	**2000**
Supply in WTE (1 Jan)[a]						
– Total (in thousands)[b]	7.9	9.7	10.7	12.2	13.9	15.3
– Active[c]	7.6	9.2	10.0	11.2	12.1	12.5
– Number providing health care[d]	7.0	8.4	9.0	10.0	11.3–10.9	12.8–11.2
– Inhabitants/WTE[e]	1405	1172	1092	984	863–891	749–858
Consumption per inhabitant per year						
Sessions						
– slow growth[f]				1.93	2.02	2.31
– rapid growth[f]	1.54	1.78	1.88	1.98	2.15	2.53
– technical services[g]	58.7	115.4	122.5			
– surgery and anesthesiology[g]	14.0	18.3	25.1			
Output per WTE						
Sessions per year[h]	2160	2103	1974	1925	1820	1895
Sessions per week[h]	48	47	44	43	41	42
Work schedule, hours per week	64–66					
Income from private work[i]						
– millions of BF (1985 prices)	2.98	3.20	2.40	2.16		

a–i See page 73.

doctors will obtain their degree) with the right to practise in Belgium (C), or this number will drop by 10% (B) or by 20% (A). The overall supply of medical graduates aged under 75 would thus reach some 39 000–40 000 in the year 2000. There would then be one medical graduate for every 235 or so inhabitants. This ratio may be impressive, but it has little significance in itself. Figure 4 provides more significant ratios per qualification and per region. In the following sections we shall attempt to forecast the future behaviour of the other components of the market up to 1990. In Sect. 3.4.4 we shall attempt to determine whether it is adviseable to maintain restrictions on medical school intake so as to be able to modify the supply situation in the year 2000.

3.3.2 Future Consumption of Health Care

Patients' consumption of health care is growing, but at a slower rate in general medicine than in specialized medicine, with respective increases of "usually" 5.3% and 8.5% per period of 5 years. Taking respective ranges of 2.5%–5% and 4.5%–8.5% per 5 years, the utilisation rates in the year 2000 could reach 5.3–6 GP sessions per inhabitant and 2.3–2.5 specialist sessions per inhabitant. For assessing the needs of new graduates, only the slow or intermediate rate of increase has been taken into account; the poor economic prospects make a quantitatively higher hypothesis less likely.

In this way, the consumption of health care by the population as a whole over the period 1974–2000 will have risen by between 11% and 26% in the case of GPs and by between 44% and 64% in the case of specialists.

The consumption figures given are the least inaccurate indicator of the demand for care in which the patient himself takes the initiative. The differing figures therefore indicate a market trend whereby consumers are gradually changing their habits and making more use of specialists, which is in line with a general trend already revealed by regional analyses.

This spontaneous tend obviously encourages an increased availablity of specialists. Consequently, the rates of growth in consumption and in manpower are very close to one

---

[a] Full-time equivalents (FTE) for MDs under 75 years old. About 200 MDs practising dental care are excluded until 1985, included from 1990 on.

[b] For 1990 and 2000: 40% practise as specialists; Scenario "A", i.e. minus 20% of new graduates from 1992 on.

[c] For 1990 and 2000: active MDs according to 1985 activity rates.

[d] For 1990 and 2000: 1985 activity rates and decreasing rates.

[e] Denominator = FTE for curative care only (ambulatory *and* hospital care).

[f] Low evolution and usual trends observed in the past.

[g] In "K" unities (K being a key index of the list of tariffs).

[h] Low hypothesis for utilisation rates. For the supply: scenario A and active MDs in curative care (ambul. for GPs; ambul plus hospital care for specialists); decreasing trend for activity rates. High hypothesis for utilization rates (trends observed in the past). For the supply: scenario A; same MDs, but 1985 activity rates. NB: If both estimates are similar, only the average is mentioned.

[i] Income stated for income tax; includes only activity as self-employed, after deduction of professional cost, but before tax (only 56% of the specialists are concerned). Source: *National Institute of Statistics.*

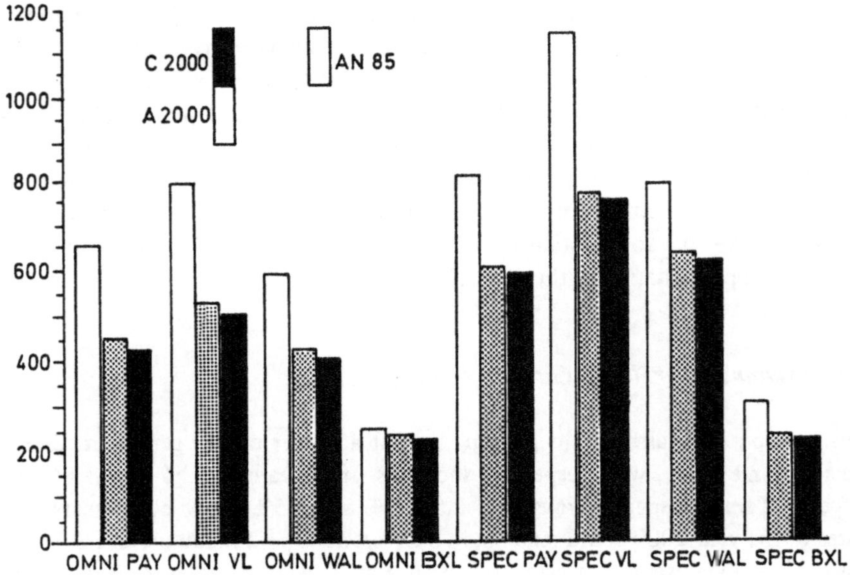

Fig. 4. Inhabitants per medical graduate (total under 75 years of age). *AN 85,* ratio for 1985; *A 2000,* ratio for 2000 with fewer graduates after 1992 (20% lower than stabilisation); *C 2000,* ratio for 2000 with a stable number of graduates. *OMNI,* general practioners; *SPEC,* specialists; *PAY,* country; *VL,* Flanders; *WAL,* Wallonia; *BXL,* Brussels

another (see Fig. 3). Moreover, there is a positive correlation between the specialist-population ratios and the level of consumption of their services (except in Flanders where these relationships are blurred by patients going from one district to another). If restrictions are placed on the number of specialists, it will be necessary to estimate their probable effect on consumption levels in both specialized and general medicine. In general medicine, the two phenomena have become independent, since here consumption is rising only slowly despite the considerable increase in manpower.

3.3.3 Future Workload

3.3.3.1 Output in Terms of Sessions

General Practitioners

Since supply and consumption have developed at very different rates, output has inevitably tended to fall (Fig. 5). In the case of GPs providing health care, annual output will fall from 7900 sessions per WTE in 1974 to 4000–5000 in 1990 and 2000, equivalent to an average drop of between 40% and 50% per WTE. Between 1974 and 1985, a drop of 37% has already occurred, and a further drop can be expected unless the specialisation rate increases.

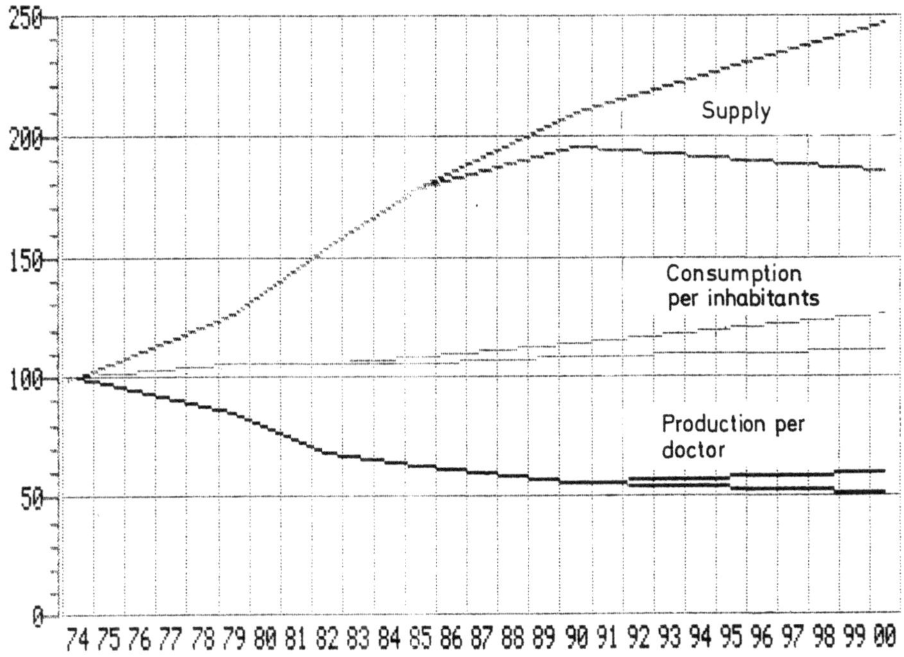

Fig. 5. Development in general practice 1974–2000: supply of active manpower, consumption per inhabitant, and output per doctor

Specialists

Average output will not vary significantly. Thus, it is anticipated that there will be a drop in the number of sessions per specialist active in health care (WTE) of about 16% between 1974 and 1990. However, most of this drop has already occurred and there will be little change between now and 2000, unless the specialization rate increases.

Calculated *per day or per week,* the above relationships take on a greater significance. Thus, GPs will see less than 100 patients per working week (compared with 175 in 1974) and specialists, some 41 per week (compared with 48 in 1974).

It should be pointed out that these output figures are calculated in terms of WTE. Consequently, the average number of patients seen by qualified doctors who provide health care during only some of their working hours will be lower. It is not clear whether these output levels are or will be sufficient to allow all doctors to maintain their skills at an adequate level; neither is it clear whether they will guarantee a range of diagnosis that is sufficiently wide to avoid mistakes when rare cases occur. However, we consider 97 patients per weeks as an acceptable productivity norm for GPs, according to ways of practice prevailing in Belgium in 1985. In regions in which averages are lower, we consider the difference as an indicator of "hidden unemployment" due to prevailing glut (5% in Wallonia). We therefore exclude 5% of the active manpower in the regions concerned before applying the "coefficient of increase of need" in order to assess the future requirements of manpower.

Table 11. Trends in the scope for hospital work

	Beds per specialist[a] Ratio	Index		
1966	7.76	100		
1974	6.82	88	100	
1981	6.06	78	89	
1990[b]	5.2–4.0	67–52	76–59	86–66

[a] Specialist: WTE engaged in health care
[b] Assumptions (1987–1990): Changes in the number of beds of +5%, –5% and –15%
Changes in the number of specialists of 20% to +30%

3.3.3.2 Derived Demand and Hospital Work

The work performed by specialists must be described in greater detail, since their total workload includes not only meetings with patients but also derived demand and hospital work.

In fact, specialists deal with (and benefit from) almost all derived demand, the volume of which they can affect in order to conform with the methods of 'modern' practice. Since modern methods introduce increasing technical sophistication to the care provided, they raise the unwritten standards of 'good practice' and, hence, the number of activities required.

A regional analysis confirms that there is a high correlation between the number of technical examinations and the number of times specialists see patients or the proportion of total health care dispensed by specialists (0.60–0.85 in 1974, depending on the region concerned); however, the correlation with the specialist-population ratio is lower (0.30–0.50) and is gradually disappearing in Flanders.

As regards hospital work, it represents a substantial part, but not all of the work performed by specialists. An analysis of work schedules and of work places shows that hospital work on average takes up half of their working time or of an 'average' load expressed in WTE. Consequently, a reduction in the scope for hospital work is not the only factor to be considered when assessing trends in specialists' workloads.

The scope for hospital work can be expressed in terms of 'beds per specialist'. The scope for such work between now and 1990 will depend on (a) the probable growth in specialist numbers, i.e. by 15%–20%; and (b) various assumptions regarding the number of hospital beds (or the total number of days spent in hospital for which refunds can be claimed). The trend is shown in Table 11, which indicates: (a) a steady reduction in the scope for hospital work by as much as 50% over a quarter of a century;[1] (b) a substantial change already seen in 1981 over 1974 (–12%) and 1966 (–22%).

It should be noted, however, that with the indicator chosen, no account can be taken in changes in treatment methods. A number of advances in diagnosis and treatment require more extensive medical work and, hence, an increase in medical staff.

Although the figures show a marked reduction in the output of non-hospital sessions and in the scope for hospital work, they can be evaluated only if other factors such as weekly output and work shedules are taken into account.

Table 12. The outlook of work schedule for specialists in 1990

	Situation in 1974 (h)	Reduction (%)		Forecast for 1990 (h)
Non-hospital work:	22–21 h	(2–14)	=	21.5–18 h
Hospital work:	24–23 h	(23–41)	=	18.5–14 h
Other activities:	20 h	(unchanged or –25%)	=	20 –15 h
Total				60 –47 h

3.3.4 Future Work Schedules

Estimates have been produced of doctors' work schedules from surveys of their work and from regional consumption statistics. Work schedules in 1990 can be estimated by applying the reducing coefficients similar to those characterizing trends in the output of doctor/patient sessions and in the volume of hospital work.

3.3.4.1 General Practitioners

Around 1990, the active general practitioner (expressed in WTE's) will work only between 34 and 40 hours, of which between 27 and 32 hours will be devoted to health care. If it is thought that the amount of work not devoted to health care should not be reduced proportionately but remain unchanged, the overall working time would be between 41 and 46 hours per week.

Expressed in these terms, the hours worked by the average general practitioner in 1990 still appear quite 'normal' and will, in fact, produce a workload which is likely to be more acceptable to him and his family.

On the other hand, the time actually worked may exceed the last estimate since GPs' greater availability may lead to an increase in the average contact time, which was about 18 minutes per session in French-speaking regions in 1971 and about 15 minutes per session in Flemish-speaking regions in 1974.

3.3.4.2 Specialists

The outlook for 1990 is shown in Table 12. Even if the number of training places settles at its present level, and despite the drastic reductions in access to hospital beds, specialists will still work a large number of hours, many more than those worked by GPs and by other members of the community.

3.3.5 How Are "Departures" To Be Interpreted?

As stated earlier, there has been a rise in the number of 'non-active' doctors. How is this trend to be interpreted? If such 'departures' are voluntary, then they are the result of personal wishes. If not, they may be caused by various strains on the market; such a hypothesis is sustained by the fact that inactivity rates are higher (a) among GPs as compared with specialists and (b) among French-speaking GPs as compared with Flemish-speaking ones: 11.8% and 8.3% under 60 years of age (compared with 6.7% for specialists), 5% being considered "normal" even when there are shortages of doctors. The differences with the rates mentioned above (the undue inactivity) may be considered as a valuable indicator of glut. The various levels of undue inactivity match perfectly with the data, concerning workload (higher for specialists) and medical demography (more densely staffed in French-speaking regions).

3.3.6 Incomes

Although income trends are not a criterion of 'needs', data on such trends may constitute a useful additional source of information.

Compared with 1973, declared incomes are falling, with a drop of 30% in the case of GPs and one of 14% in the case of specialists (at constant prices).[6] Despite this drop, these incomes are still more than adequate and remain among the highest recorded for self-employed professional people. Thus, medical specialists are in first place (BF 2.08 million in 1984), followed by notaries (BF 1.96 million), general practitioners (BF 1.33 million) and pharmacists (BF 1.30 million).

Such averages conceal large regional variations, reaching almost 1 to 2: for GPs, BF 0.88 million in Brussels, BF 1.24 million in Wallonia and BF 1.55 million in Flanders; for specialists, BF 1.19 million in Brussels, BF 1.97 million in Wallonia and BF 2.35 million in Flanders.

Even among young doctors, the situation is not as catastrophic as might have been thought, since their average incomes in 1981 were BF 700 000 for GPs and BF 1.5 million for young specialists. However, a significant proportion of doctors earn relatively little from their private work, one-third of GPs and one-fifth of specialists declaring less than BF 500 000. This category probably includes doctors performing work for part of the year, such as those who recently settle a practice or who retire or die during the year, as well as specialists who combine a private practice with a salaried hospital post.

3.3.7 Factors Influencing Requirements of Medical Manpower

A number of factors influencing requirements of medical manpower can be identified; most indicate an upward trend.

3.3.7.1 Factors Affecting Consumption

The *ageing* of the population increases needs. Between 1985 and the year 2000, the percentage of persons aged 65 or over in Belgium will increase from 14% to 17% and, as is well known, the health-care consumption of this age-group is greater than that of other adults.

---

6 Source for incomes here and ff., Institut National de Statistique (Income from *private* work only, before tax but minus professional expenses).

Medical advances enable more chronically ill and handicapped persons, who have a high health-care consumption, to be kept alive.

The *adverse effects* of industrialization show little sign of decreasing; there are increased feelings of insecurity owing, for example, to unemployment and changes in working practices (which are known to cause illness) resulting from the development of micro-electronics and the world recession.

The desire of the public authorities to standardize behaviour with a view to improving health will lead to a type of *hypersurveillance* (to use J. Attali's expression), and this will generate increased consumption.

Awareness of illness and the *desire for health care* are increasing; this results from imitation, a desire to conform to a general norm, from 'self-observation' (which induces anxiety), and from a new taste for "non-classical" types of therapy, e.g. homeopathy, accupuncture.

On the other hand, the *desire to reduce public expenditure* will tend to put pressure on the amounts refunded to patients and on the services paid for by the insurance schemes, which will this reintroduce an economic constraint on access to health care, especially in low-income groups.

Over the longer term, this acute problem in the financing of health care might be resolved by an *output stimulus* resulting from a change in health-care patterns, in which

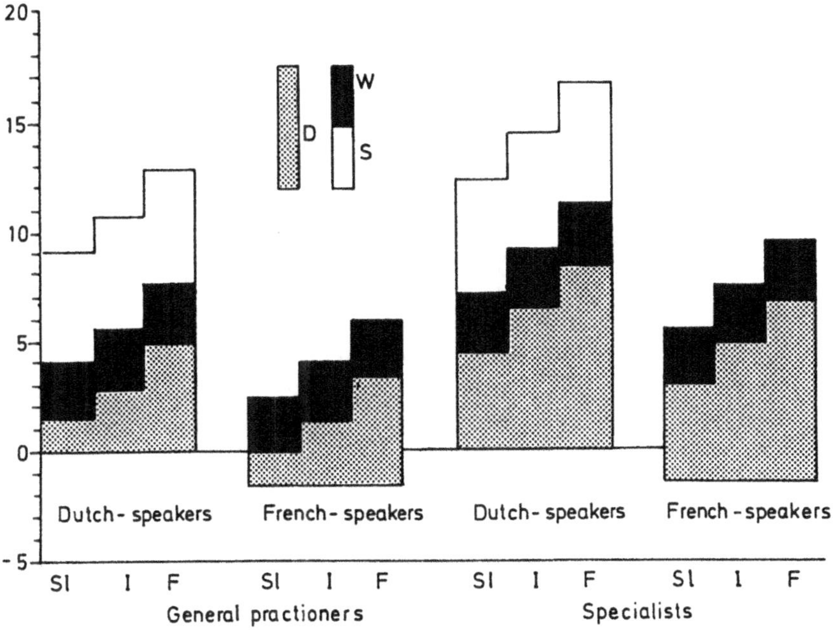

Fig. 6. Development of requirements of medical manpower (percentage growth every 5 years). *D*, demand (negative growth reflects the impact of a reduction in the population); *W*, work: reduction in hours of work (2.5% per 5-year period); *S*, share: share in the work (5% per 5-year period); *Sl*, slow rate of growth; *I*, intermediate rate of growth, similar to the past; *F*, fast rate of growth

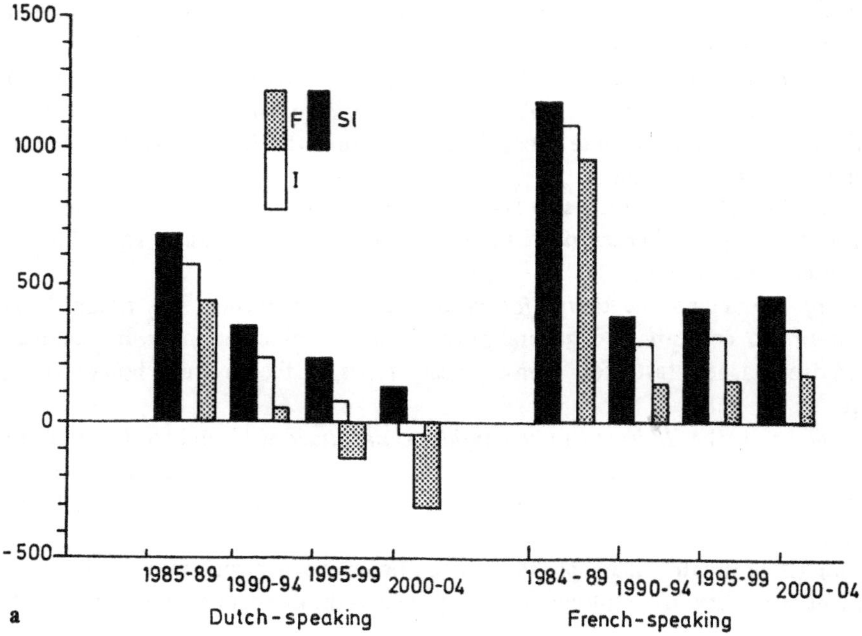

a

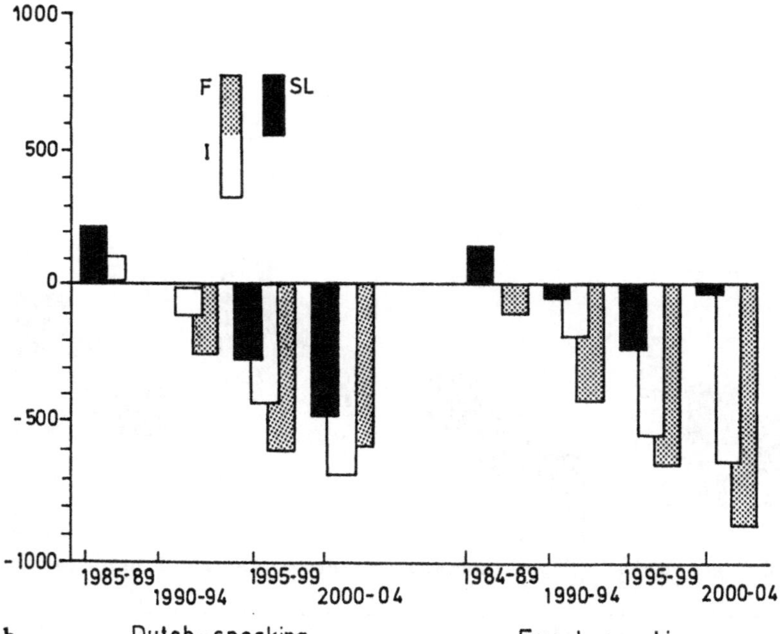

b

Fig. 7a, b. Excess of supply of active medical graduates over ideal requirements: 5-year analysis. **a** General practitioners. Note: These figures are based on a hypothesis which assumes stability in the numbers of non-active doctors over the age of 60 (scenario dC). It is probable that the excess of supply will in fact encourage a higher rate of non-activity than predicted by this hypothesis. **b** Specialists. Note: The effective shortages will probably be smaller as the figures for specialisation rise above 40%. *Sl, I, F,* see legend to Fig. 6

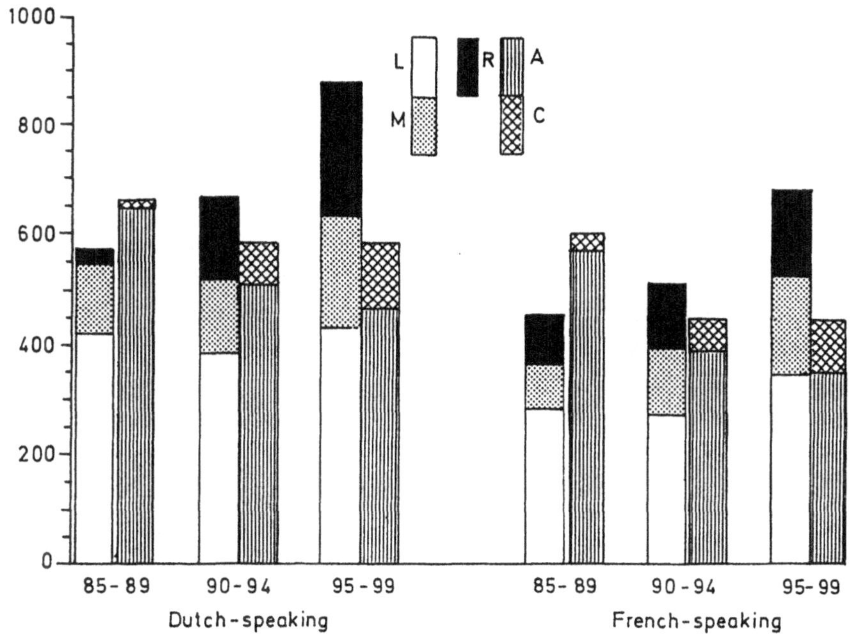

Fig. 8. Annual requirements and expected levels of graduates. Requirements: *Sl, I, F,* see legend to Fig. 6. Supply: *C,* number of graduates stabilising at the level reached in 1992; *A,* 20% less than *C*

diagnostic equipment, long-distance consultations, medical computers and computer programs, and prosthetic devices would be made available for public consumption.

3.3.7.2 Factors Affecting Medical Practice

The *scope* of medicine is widening, partly at the expense of other professions and partly under the impact of technical progress (e.g. in bioingeneering).

The *demographic characteristics* of the medical profession are changing: thus, women make up an increasing proportion of the medical profession and will continue to work, albeit for fewer hours (45 hours per week in 1971) than their male counterparts (60 hours per week in 1971).

The *doctor's working life* might become shorter; in 1977, the register of the Department for Socioeconomic Studies in the Health Field Louvain University showed that 90% of doctors in the 65–74 age group were still active; in 1983, this figure had dropped to 68%; if such a trend continues, the percentage of active doctors above 65 years of age might drop to 23% in the year 2000.

Working hours are being reduced in all occupations; it is unlikely that young doctors will want (or be able) to continue working an average of 60 hours per week, as they did in 1971.

Average output per doctor has been falling since 1974; not only does this affect the total amount of time worked; at the same time, the average length of doctor-patient sessions might increase, which affects the balance between supply and demand.

3.3.8 Assessing Future Requirements

We have now identified a dozen factors which will definitely affect the demands of the general population and the conditions under which doctors work in the years to come. Several assumptions can be made regarding the way in which each of these factors is likely to evolve in the next 10 years. In each case further assumptions may then be made regarding the impact of these changes on the number of doctors 'required'. If these various assumptions, all equally plausible, are combined, the result is a set of possibilities which comprise several hundred situations. Under these circumstances, the traditional question regarding the number of doctors needed cannot be given a clear and unambiguous answer. However, it is possible to work out certain types of needs which are indisputable and to put forward some general assumptions.

3.4 Suggested Courses of Action

In view of the present oversupply and of the forecasts of growth, and bearing in mind the prospect of difficult economic circumstances and of limitations on public spending, what manpower policies can be considered? The key questions are as follows:

- How can the available manpower best be used?
- How can a better geographical distribution be encouraged?
- Must access to posts in specialized medicine be restricted?
- Must medical school intakes be limited?

3.4.1 Using Available Manpower

In view of the influx of medical graduates, various questions have to be asked:

- How can new activities of value to public health be promoted?
- How can a situation be brought about in which the available work is distributed among a larger number of doctors?
- How can expenditure, rather than manpower, be controlled?

3.4.1.1 New Prospects?

Since, in general, the supply of curative health care in Belgium is satisfactory, are there other sectors where needs have not yet been met?

Preventive community medicine, health education, research, and epidemiology would almost certainly benefit from having more medical staff. It is to a large extent up to the public authorities to make the requisite funds available. It is also up to doctors and hospitals to take advantage of the extraordinary potential of medical informatics, which can contribute significantly to epidemiology, pharmco-vigilance, and medical research, assist in determining diagnosis and treatment, and help to give a scientific foundation to planning for equipment and services. In day-to-day work, the computer will become an indispensable means of obtaining access to comprehensive information which is continuously being updated, of assessing one's own working methods, and of evaluating the success or failure of various treatments by comparing them with overall data. New posts for such useful work could thus be promoted, but availability of public funding will be scarce.

Medical assistance to the Third World offers a vast range of potential work opportunities to doctors. The needs are immense: whole continents have only one doctor for every 10 000 or more inhabitants. Admittedly, these needs cannot always be met and, moreover, the available infrastructure is very inadequate. However, there is no lack of young, energetic doctors ready to go to these countries, on condition that they are guaranteed a job, the requisite facilities when they arrive and, above all, some job security when they return home. It would be advantageous if the ad hoc bodies concerned had sufficient resources so that they could do more to determine the need for, and promote, development projects and cooperation agreements, improve the information given to young doctors, and find original solutions to the problem of the status of development aid workers; thus, doctors do not necessarily have to receive the standard 'international' salary, but perhaps they can be given reintegration assistance to overcome the problems frequently encountered when returning home. It might be possible, for example, to find posts in the public service for doctors who have worked for 15 or 20 years in the Third World. However, such a project does not necessarily meet the wishes of the Third World: they have more immediate needs and they prefer medical treatment to be provided by natives, in accordance with the development principle of attempting to achieve self-reliance. Furthermore, working in developing countries is a job requiring specific motivation; it is possible for a limited number of doctors. However, it is not the proper way for the industrialised countries to "get rid" of their oversupply.

3.4.1.2 Work Sharing

The question of work and income sharing has to be faced by all workers and governments, owing to the rise in unemployment which is occurring in every European country and in every employment sector. Medicine is one of the areas affected. The following steps could be taken to deal with the problem:

- *The retirement of doctors at 65* should be encouraged and subsequently made compulsory under a mutual medical insurance agreement. Forbidding elderly doctors to work might not be necessary, but the refunding scheme operated by the INAMI (National Institute for Sickness and Disability Insurance) could be changed or reduced in scope. This will be acceptable to doctors only of they can be guaranteed an adequate pension. If applied generally from 1985 onwards, this measure would make available 2000–3400 posts over 5 years depending on when it is put into force but would have little or no effect over the subsequently.
- *Working both in hospitals and in private practice* should be discouraged by making it easier for specialists to work in a single hospital, if possible on a full-time basis and

without a practice elsewhere. The possibility of giving consultations in several private practices should be limited to justified cases, with a maximum of two practices per doctor.

- An attempt should be made to draw up *guidelines regarding the number of medical staff required in hospitals.* The nature, scale and equipment of the services concerned should be borne in mind, in particular to maintain the quality of health care and to ensure that the staff can work in safe conditions. This could counteract the currently existing monopolistic situations which hamper the recruitment of additional staff.
- *The average number of patients seen or sessions held* each year by any one doctor should be limited so as to improve the quality of work in regions where work is still very intensive, and to share work among the whole of the medical profession. Any measure of this kind would have to respect the doctor's freedom to choose the appropriate treatment and the patient's right to choose which doctor he sees: the main objective is not necessarily incompatible with these fundamental principles. Certain measures already adopted move in this direction: the duty to record the amount received in professional fees will make tax evasion more difficult and thus discourage very high output.
- In view of the increased competition from specialists and the encroaching of specialists on the traditional role of the general practitioner, particularly in urban areas, it might be useful to promote the *general practitioner's general role* and his coordinating function between preventive and curative health care. It will probably also be necessary to encourage a system whereby each person would be compelled to enrol on a GPs list or to consult him before meeting a specialist.

3.4.1.3 Controlling Expenditures Rather than Supply

The sharp rise in expenditures for the provision of technical services, due in particular to an expansion in the supply of specialized doctors inevitably casts doubt on the advisability of refunding the cost of these services on a fee for service basis, especially when the increasing automatization of the production process is leading to an enormous rise in productivity. If technological progress is to be harnessed without leading to the collapse of the sickness insurance system, a new financing system should be worked out. As is done in some hospital budgets, the fixed expenses of the centres authorized to provide technical services could be covered at their actual cost, and only variable costs would be reimbursed in proportion to the number of treatments given. This proposal, which we have been putting forward since 1980, is now being carefully examined by the Government and, if adopted, it will supplement a number of measures which have already been taken to limit expenditures (see Sect. 2.2.3).[7]

---

7 There are several alternatives, including a control on the number of patients' health record cards, a special contribution to be paid by overprescribers (possibly redistributed among underdescribers), or smaller refunds for patients who go to doctors with a very high output. Since solutions of this kind have not yet been tried, each one should be carefully assessed in terms of its potential advantages and disadvantages before it is put up for negotiation or applied.

3.4.2 Improving Geographical Distribution

Bringing in an 'establishment law' that would lay down in an authoritarian way rules governing where doctors can set up practice does not appear to be an adequate solution to the problem. It would seem more sensible to provide more information so that manpower can be directed in a flexible way, depending on the 'relative needs' of the population.

3.4.2.1 An Unjustifiable Solution: An Establishment Law

Paradoxically, schemes for the compulsory distribution of doctors are being put forward at a time when they are less required than they have ever been. Contrary to the situation in the past, the gradual saturation of the market is inducing young doctors to look more than they used to for those areas most likely to provide a potential clientele, irrespective of the residential considerations that once guided a doctor's choice. For the first time the interest of young doctors coincide with those of the population.

In addition, introducing an establishment law would involve serious risks, with consequences worse than the current freedom of action. It would also come up against technical difficulties. Some of these could be overcome, but there is one basic objection: There is no objective basis for compulsory standards.

The Risks

1. Any error in drawing up the standards would only perpetuate distorsions, whereas free-market forces would immediately correct any individual errors made.
2. Any standard would fail to meet the local needs of a number of areas with poor medical services that happen to be within larger regions with extremely good medical coverage.
3. Holding back the renewal of medical practice, which is desirable in view of the continual changes which are occurring, by permanently fixing the areas where doctors can practise and by introducing a system of control by elderly colleagues, would cause medicine to become much less dynamic.
4. Social injustice would result if young doctors who have trained for between 7 and 15 years were prevented from working, were obliged to work as employees for doctors who already had a practice, or were forced clandestinely and at increasing cost to purchase from retiring doctors the right to care for their usual patients.
5. There would be a greater temptation to increase output in order to pay for these clandestine 'purchases' and to make up for the low salary received when working as an employee. The limitation of supply would thus provide no effective limitation on consumption.
6. There would be high-handedness and sectarian conflicts, even abuses and corruption, in the absence of any irrefutable objective standards.

The Technical Difficulties

Both requirements and supply are difficult to measure.

1. Requirements are an ambiguous concept. Epidemiological data and assessments of their implications in terms of the number of doctors required do not yet exist at a national level, let alone at a regional level. All that can be cone is to refer to the 'levels of con-

sumption', although these have to be adjusted according to age-group distribution. When linked to the doctor-population ratio, consumption levels can undoubtedly provide a useful indication of 'workload', but they cannot be a basis for compulsory standards.

2. Figures showing the *supply* of doctors must reflect how doctors actually work, and must be broken down according to the various places of work. However they may be well kept, official registers normally fulfil other aims and are thus unsuitable as a basis of policy-making. Limited by their own subjectives and by administrative constraints, they do not permit an adequate analysis of the real health-care market. Updating them involves the slow transmission of data through different hierarchical levels, and they usually yield only a single address for each doctor, without any gurantee that any medical work is being carried out there. In order to measure regional supply they would have to be extensively modified, as would the rules for recording, transmitting and coding information on medical work.

Absence of Standards

The problem may not be tackled, by comparing doctor-population ratios in line with the criteria used for pharmacies and for hospital planning. The simplicity of such a solution is appealing, but sumplicity is poor criterion in this particular case. There are no valid grounds for aggregating average doctor-to-population ratios, regardless of whether these concern all doctors or individual groups of specialists.

How should geographical units be selected? In the case of GPs the administrative units are too large, while in specialized medicine no one unit is really adequate, owing to the gravitational pull exercised by hospitals; in addition, the radius within which doctors work varies from one speciality to another.

The implicit assumption that doctor-population ratios should be evened out is erroneous for the following reasons: (a) The introdcution of more doctors in certain areas with a small number of doctors does not always meet a 'need' felt by the population, who may remain low consumers of health care, as has been shown by our studies; (b) in specialized medicine, a certain proportion of consumption must remain centred on large inter-regional hospitals; account must also be taken of possible overlapping between specialities.

From a scientific as well as from a political point of view, it is unrealistic to believe that the organisations involved can establish objective standards for the various specialities, taking into account the multifaceted relationships between supply, consumption and need, as well as the scale of the hospital infrastructure and the geographical area covered by each speciality. Leaving the decisions to national or regional committees might open the way to all kinds of political intrigue, while in no may improving public health, the finances of sickness insurance schemes or access to medical care.

3.4.2.2 The Proposed Solution: Information to Guide Doctors

Decentralized Information Services

Although it is not adviseable to even out doctor-population ratios on a general basis, improved distribution can be sought by means of a flexible and effective information system available to doctors looking for an area in which to practise. A system of this kind has been successfully operating in Belgium for several years; it was initially set up in the Department for Socioeconomic Studies in the Health Field at the Catholic University of Louvain and is available for all students and doctors.

The experience thus gained shows that young doctors do intend to examine the 'relative needs' of the population so as to maximize their changes of finding patients in spite of the gradual saturation of the market. A service of this kind is also in the interests of potential clients and avoids the rigidity of a compulsory 'establishment law'; the information is given for guidance purposes only and can be freely interpreted on the basis of various criteria and compared with the existing situation, which changes from day to day.

If all doctors are provided with adequate, objective information, the market becomes more transparent. The enterprising spirit and ingenuity of doctors using such an instrument should produce an acceptable geographical distribution of manpower in a much more reliable way than standards based on a mathematical model which, however sophisticated, inevitably involves imprecise parameters and a multiplicity of assumptions.

In fact, a system of this kind has been officially tested in France. In June 1977, the Minister of Health and Family Affairs asked the Regional Directorate for Health and Social Affairs in Aquitaine to prepare and test a methodology for establishing information centres for doctors and medical students. This scheme was designed to meet the urgent need for information on the part of doctors and medical students looking for an area in which to practise, and to 'improve overall knowledge of medical demography at relatively fine levels of geographical breakdown'. Wherever possible, information should be at the level of individual municipalities and not regionally based. This is because a 'relative need', i.e. an area in which the supply of doctors is somewhat less abundant, can now be identified only at a local level. The following information should be available.

Type of Information Provided

Supply of Health Care (see Appendix 1 for characteristics of the basic register).

- Doctor-population ratios and the number of potential patients per doctor, by district and municipality, according to (a) medical qualification: GPs, specialists by speciality; (b) type of activity: non-hospital treatment, hospital treatment, other activities including preventive medicine.
- Age structure of the medical profession: broken down by speciality, district and municipality.

Consumption of Health Care. The rates are given by district and by type of health care; the overall scope for working in a given area depends on the level of health-care consumption.

'Average Output'. This is expressed as the number of sessions per physician, and indices are given for each district. These statistics indicate the average workload in response to patients' requests; if the load is high, it demonstrates the existence of a demand which could be distributed more easily over a larger number of doctors.

Sociodemographic Characteristics of the Municipalities

- Population density: In rural areas, greater distances have to be travelled for house calls.
- Demographic change: An expanding area offers better job prospects.
- Age structure of the population: A high proportion of elderly persons indicates that the 'need' for health care is relatively high.

Method of Guidance

A guidance centre is neither an employment office nor a body specializing in market studies. The applicant must therefore make his or her own decision in the light of the information provided. Moreover, GPs and specialists must use this information in different ways.

A *general practitioner* who is prepared to practise anywhere should rely mainly on the figures for 'average output': in places where they exceed the average for the area considered it will be easier to set up practice, because it should be easier for the existing demand to be spread over a larger number of doctors. If doctors choose a specific subregion, they should look for a suitable municipality or district within it. If there is no information on consumption at this level, they will have to compare doctor-population ratios, also taking account of the demographic characteristics of the population and of doctors: thus, 800 inhabitants per general practitioner apparently becomes the maximal level for which a location can still be found in Belgium, but no guarantee can be provided that such a size is still viable. If there is still uncertainty, it would be useful to obtain additional information so as to identify those areas where elderly doctors will reduce their workload or cease working altogether in the next few years.

The doctors concerned should also look at the presence of specialists and the consumption of specialized medicine so as to assess potential competition. In addition, they should look at recent population trends (indicating whether a municipality is expanding or declining) and at the proportion of elderly persons in the population (indicating a greater need).

Specialists often work in a hospital or in collaboration with a hospital. Here, personal relationships are of crucial importance. However, some specialists request information on the regional distribution of specialists. If a doctor is looking for a hospital post, figures relating the number of specialists to the number of ad hoc hospital beds will certainly show the gaps existing at the regional level and will help to guide his search; however, the final decision is not made by him, since it is necessary to convince both the specialist in charge of the department and the hospital management that he is needed. Personal contact therefore remains essential. As regards setting up a private practice, specialists will be given the same information on their speciality as that prepared for general practitioners (with the exception of average output). It will have to be used with greater care, since the various field of work overlap (particularly in internal medicine) and the size of the area on which they can draw differs from one speciality to another. If local supply does not appear to meet demand, a specialist setting up practice in a particular district may be able to meet part of the local demand.

If there is no doctor in a particular district who specializes in a certain field and if the demand for that speciality is low, demand may increase if the opening of a new practice facilitates access to the type of care required.

3.4.3 Should the Number of Specialists Be Limited?

In view of the growth in the number of doctors and the restrictions of hospital building, the "Conseil supérieur des medécins spécialistes" (Board of Medical Specialists) is proposing that restrictions be placed in future on the number of trainee-specialists.

How desirable are these plans from the point of view of young doctors and planners? Unless other planning requirements indicate the contrary, it might be useful to start by examining the criterion of *"workload"*. As indicated in Sect. 3.3, the different rates of growth in consumption (more rapid in specialized medicine) and in manpower (much lower in specialized medicine) will lead to (a) a steady drop in the workload of GPs and (b) a stabilization in the workload of specialists at a level involving a high number of hours worked per week, despite the large drop which will occur in the number of hospital beds per specialist.

Consequently, planners must examine the advisability of a policy restricting the number of specialists in the light of public interest. Their decision will affect health policies, the control of public expenditure and the employment of young doctors.

As regards *public health*, are such measures likely to shift the balance of the health system towards primary health care, as advocated by international bodies? In practice, this type of care will not benefit at all from the measures proposed. Other steps need to be taken to promote this type of care, particularly those designed to assist the coordination of health care between various types of medical staff.

As regards *public expenditure*, the growth in the supply of specialists would probably lead to an increase in specialized, technical treatments, as has been observed in the past, and hence to further upward pressure on expenditure for health care. However, there is no guarantee that imposing a limit on the number of specialists will actually halt the growth in the use of technology and in the attendant costs.

It will therefore be necessary to take back-up measures, some of which have already been mentioned in Sect. 3.4.1:

- Overall budget ceilings for hospitals
- Laboratories to operate within a budget covering fixed costs, with variable costs being covered at an average rate
- Controlling the amount of technical treatments prescribed, with financial incentives promoting moderate uses of the resources in the health system

If they were taken, measures of this kind might make it less necessary to limit the number of specialists, because if output is controlled there will be room for more young doctors, given the probable activity and income levels.

The *concern about the employment of young doctors* should therefore induce the planner not to restrict the number of specialists. In fact, a substantial increase is acceptable on condition that ad hoc back-up measures are taken to control public expenditure. There is even a threat of shortage in the future, if the rate of specialisation remains as low as 40%. The level of acceptable growth should be laid down for each speciality, with account taken of the relevant age structure as well as of forecasts regarding the amount of disease requiring treatment and the types of treatment available. At all events, the distribution of work among doctors should be facilitated by a measure already mentioned above, namely the introduction of minimum hospital staffing levels depending on the nature and size of the department concerned.

3.4.4 Advisability of Restricting Medical School Intake

Since 1973 our team has argued in favour of limiting the number of medical students. However, now that the number of students beginning medical studies has dropped dramatically, is it advisable to advocate a measure of this kind? A measure of self-regulation appears to have occurred already, and applying a further brake might make it less easy in the future to meet the growing needs of the population.

Denmark

J.P. Steensen

1 The Danish Health Service

1.1 Population and Administration

Denmark has a population of 5.1 million inhabitants. The population total has stabilized in the last decade, and the substantial elements in demographic development at the present time are a low birth rate and an increase in the elderly population.

Geographically, the country is divided by the Great Belt (*Store Baelt*). Approximately 45% of the population is concentrated in the eastern region , which includes the capital area, and this part of the country is the most urbanized. In the western region, the population is a mixture of rural and urban inhabitants. The two most important population concentrations in this region are the university towns of Aarhus and Odense.

Administratively, the country is divided into 16 counties with an average of 300000 inhabitants per county. It is also divided into 275 municipalities whose sizes vary from a couple of thousand inhabitants to half a million in the capital.

The Faeroe Islands and Greenland, in the North Atlantic, which have a total population of approximately 80 000 are in federation with Denmark.

1.2 Organization of the Health Service

One of the priorities for the organization of the health service is to ensure for all citizens, regardless of geographical location and income, open and equal access to doctor and hospital treatment. The health service includes both public and private elements, but any private sectors costs to citizens are more or less covered by a health insurance scheme.

The primary health service covers a range of independent professionals, such as general practitioners (GPs) and dentists, who are associated with the Health Insurance Scheme. It also attends to various special functions in local communities, e.g. child dental care and district nurse services.

The hospital service is publicly financed and includes a number of hospitals differing in size and specialization. Organization of the hospital service must ensure a geographical distribution of facilities, whilst offering the possibility of highly specialized treatment.

The management and administration of the health service are decentralized. The most important units are the County Councils, which administer both the hospital services and the Health Insurance Scheme. The public functions of the primary health service, other than the Health Insurance Scheme, are dealt with by the municipalities.

The government's obligations in connection with the health service relate to supervision and control of medical personnel and institutions. The government is also involved in the ultimate planning and distribution of resources.

The actual form of organization in the various sections of the health service is historically determined. The Health Insurance Scheme has evolved from a private health scheme, whilst the hospital service has always been in the public sector. The direct public functions of the primary health service were established much later, in a period when health service was generally considered to be a public function.

1.3 The Primary Health Service

The tasks of the municipalities in the primary health service cover health visitors, child dental care, the school medical service and district nurse services. They are managed and administered by the individual local authorities in conjunction with other public services provided by local communities, e.g. schools and social services.

The task of the counties in the primary health service is the running of the Health Insurance Scheme, which includes GPs, practising specialists, dentists, practising physiotherapists and other health personnel. The Health Insurance Scheme also administers the government's subsidy to medicine.

There are two categories of Health Insurance, and citizens can choose the category to which they wish to belong. Category 1, which accounts for 95% of the population, gives free access to examination and treatment by GPs and specialists. It also provides a subsidy for dental care, physiotherapy and medicine. Category 1 patients are assigned to a GP in their area, from whom a recommendation is required for specialist treatment.

It is possible to change one's doctor once a year. Category 2 patients can choose GP for each visit and specialist treatment is available to them without a GP's recommendation. However, the Health Insurance Scheme only refunds part of the cost of any medical treatment. The percentage of catagory 2 patients, most of whom live in the larger towns, has decreased.

General practice is a corner-stone of the health service. It is a family doctor system in which, generally speaking, there is patient-doctor contact over a number of years, and it is well developed in all areas of the country, with one GP to approximately 1700–1800 inhabitants. Ninety per cent of all consultations are delt with entirely by the GPs themselves. At the same time, general practice is "a filter" for the specialized health service in that access to specialists and hospitals is normally the result of a recommendation from a GP.

The Health Insurance Scheme is administered and regulated by means of legislation and agreements between the Health Insurance authorities and the various professional organizations. Regulations cover the setting of fees, the number of practising doctors and their geographical distribution. They are most comprehensive with regard to doctors and to the distribution of medicines, but it is also in those spheres that the authorities' economic involvement is greatest.

1.4 The Hospital Service

Hospitals are owned and run by the counties, and the highest authority in each county is the County Council, which is comprised of politicians. The number of hospitals, their size and their degree of specialization are decided by the individual County Council after consultation with the Ministry of the Interior.

There are 125 hospitals in all, with a total of approximately 40 000 beds. The hospital structure is, in principle, divided into three parts. Local hospitals account for a few departments and have a very fluctuating population. Central hospitals exist in all County Council areas and have an average of 15 different specialist departments and supply a population of approximately 200 000. Regional hospitals have all the specialist facilities and supply a population of one million.

The consumption of hospital resources is affected hospital treatment required by the population, the politically established standards of hospital treatment, and agreements with the various hospital staff unions. The County Councils decide the personnel quota in the individual hospital departments. Agreements with the unions on working hours, breaks, working areas, classification of occupations etc. have an influence, however, on the minimum quota necessary for the functioning of a hospital department.

1.5 Functions of the Government

The Ministry of the Interior is the highest health/political authority and must approve all Health Insurance agreements and hospital planning before they can be put into effect. It administers, furthermore, need-determined grants to the counties and prepares legislation for Parliament in the health/political sphere.

The National Board of Health works under the Ministry of the Interior and is run by doctors. It assists the Ministry of the Interior in the evaluation of hospital planning and the preparation of legislation, but can also – on its own initiative – consider any issue of medical importance. It is responsible for the authorization of medical personnel and implements a range of supervisory and control measures. In addition it collects information about activity and the use of resources in the health service, and about demographic statistics.

Medical officers are to be found in all counties and are the local representatives of the Ministry of the Interior and the National Board of Health.

The training of medical personnel is handled by both the government and the counties. The supreme governmental authority is the Ministry of Education, which is advised by a special committee – the National Professional Committee for Health Education – comprised of representatives from educational institutions, health authorities and the medical profession. The Committee advises the Ministry on all questions concerning the orientation of studies, admission requirements and the annual number of students entering the various health education establishments.

1.6 Expenditure and Development Trends

From the mid-1950s to the mid 1970s the health service expanded extensively in all regions of the country, and its percentage of the gross national product rose from 2% to 6% over a period of 20 years. The expansion was especially noticeable in the hospital service, and it was only at the end of this period that a certain amount of expansion in the primary health service also took place.

Since the end of the 1970s development has been substantially steadier, partly because the health service is well developed in all areas of the country and partly because there has been grater pressure to limit growth in the use of public resources. Today most of the increase in costs in the health service is due to the growing number of elderly people.

At present time there are approximately 115 000 full-time employees in the health service, 90 000 of whom are in the hospital service. The main problems are adjustment of the various functions of the health service to demographic changes and maintenance of tight control on the costs. In addition, there are attempts to shift the burden in the health service from the financially onerous hospital service to the primary health service.

2 Doctors' Training and Practice

2.1 Pregraduate Training

Medical facilities are to be found at the universities of Copenhagen, Aarhus and Odense. The average training course lasts seven years. Since 1976 admission to medical school has been limited. Fifty per cent of places are allocated to students who have the highest secondary examination grades, and 40% on basis of examination grades together with occupational experience. A certain amount of working experience can augment an examination grade that is below the average for immediate admission to medical school. The remaining 10% of places are reserved for mature students after evaluation of each application.

After a one-year study period, students must take assessment examination. On average, 80% of students pass this examination and later graduate as doctors of medicine.

The number of admissions to medical school are determined annually by the Ministry of Education after consultation with the National Professional Committee for Health Education. In assessing the number of places, forecasts regarding the supply of qualified doctors and expectations of future demand are taken into account.

A medical degree from a Danish university enables one to work as a hospital registrar or in general practice.

2.2 Postgraduate Training

Postgraduate training consists of practical clinical experience and theoretical courses. The practical side of the training comprises employment in different positions as registrar und senior registrar in the hospital service and general practice. To ensure a steady flow, all registrar and senior registrar positions have a fixed duration. All hospital departments are classified by the National Board of Health according to speciality, degree of specialization, number of beds, patient turnover, number of staff members and access to service facilities.

Postgraduate theoretical courses are organized by the National Board of Health and are given in connection with employment in certain registrar positions.

To obtain authorization to set up as a general practitioner or a specialist, it is necessary to have had experience in a number of different hospital departments and in general practice for fixed periods of time which are prescribed in detail by the National Board of Health for each speciality.

Common to all postgraduate training is an 18-month period of basic training, comprising 6 months of surgery, 6 months of internal medicine and 6 months in general practice.

GP training takes another 3 1/2 years and specialist training 4 1/2–7 years. The total training periods for authorization to set up as a GP or a specialist are 5 and 6–8 1/2 years respectively.

Admission to specialist training is regulated through registrar positions at regional hospitals. Employment in these positions is obligatory in all specialist training, and the number of vacancies in individual fields is limited. The number of registrar positions in general practice is the limiting factor for the number of doctors that can qualify for authorization to set up as a GP.

The number of medical specialities and the number of training posts for each speciality and for general practice are fixed by the Ministry of the Interior after consultation with a committee composed mostly of representatives of the public health authorities and politicians. The detailed postgraduate training programme and the issue of authorizations are dealt with by a committee composed mostly of doctors on the National Board of Health.

The postgraduate training of doctors is, in fact, based on frequent rotation and on competition for a limited number of key registrar positions which must bes secured in order to obtain authorization as a specialist or a GP. In practice, the training procedures are somewhat longer than the formal training requirements demand.

2.3 Career Progress

University training usually ends about the age of 27–28 and ist followed by the basic training, after which there is a choice between general practice or specialist training.

Authorization as a GP is usually attained 7–8 years after graduation. Establishment in general practice can take place once a practice is available. Authorization as a specialist is generally attained approximately 10 years after graduation, i.e. in one's late 30s. It is now possible to become established as a specialist when a practice becomes available, or a doctor's hospital training can continue for some years, with a view to his qualifying for the position of a medial superintendent. Appointment as a medical superintendent occurs most frequently 15 years after graduation from medical school, at about the age of 40.

The conditions for doctors in the more important sectors – registrars and medical superintendents in the hospital service, GPs and practising specialists – will be described below. The organizational relationships concerning the medical profession will also briefly described.

2.4 Hospital Doctors

The number of doctor positions in the hospital service depends first of all on the population's neeed for hospital treatment and on political decisions regarding the capacity, accessibility and degree of specialization of hospitals. Agreements on working conditions, however, have an effect on the minimum staffing necessary to operate a hospital department.

Junior doctors can be employed as registrars or senior registrars. Registrar positions are of between 1 and 3 years' duration, whereas senior registrar positions are of 5 years' duration. Working time must not exceed an average of 40–45 hours per week (including any on-call duties), at least 20 of which must be during the day. Furthermore, there are fixed limits on the maximum frequency of duty. Planning of breaks and days off are of less importance in the planning of doctor allocation in the individual hospital departments.

The number of posts for medical superintendents is regulated by means of a thorough evaluation of the need to have leading specialists in the individual departments on a regular basis. Previously, there was a staff structure arrangement which ensured a regular fixed ratio between the number of medical superintendents and the number of registrars with regard to training and experience. This arrangement has not been applied since the end of the 1970s.

2.5 General Practice

When a new doctor takes over an established practice, there is a financial transaction between the two parties. As the main source of income is from the Health Insurance Scheme, the situation is strictly regulated by means of legislative decisions in particular, by agreements between the Health Insurance Scheme and the Association of General Practitioners.

The individual practitioner is responsible for the financial and administrative aspects of the practice, subject to certain minimum requirements concerning location, consultation times and on-call duties. He can decide if he wishes to work alone or, as happens more frequently, in partnership with other doctors in a joint practice. The income from the Health Insurance Scheme must cover the running costs for the practice, as well as assistants' and doctors' salaries. The number of practitioners in an area is regulated according to the number of practitioners in an area. The aim is an even distribution of patients among the practitioners, and there is a limit to the number of patients that a practitioner may have. Approximately 50% of the income of a practice is derived from a per capita payment which is made according to the number of patients. The remaining 50% comprises fee-for-service payments. Any increase in the number of consultations necessitates the establishment of extra practices. Therefore, an increase in the number of consultations leads to the employment of more doctors rather than to higher incomes for established doctors. Regulations differ in the central parts of the capital area, where practitioners are salaried according to the number of their patients.

Conditions for practitioners are laid down by negotiations every other year between the Health Insurance Scheme and the Association of General Practitioners. Only doctors who are covered by these agreements may work for the Health Insurance Scheme. Any incidental problems concerning general practice are dealt with by a board which is composed of equal numbers of local and national practice representatives of the Health Insurance Scheme and GPs.

2.6 Practising Specialists

Specialist practice is, like general practice, a liberal profession. Its main source of income is the Health Insurance Scheme and, like general practice, it is regulated by legislation and agreements.

Practising specialists can be either part-time or full-time. Most full-time specialists are found in specialities with extensive out-patient treatment, e.g. othology, ophthalmology and psychiatry. Part-time specialists are to be found in all fields and are most often hospital medical superintendents who work a number of hours a week in specialist practice, in addition to carrying out their hospital work. Only those specialists covered by the agreement between the Health Insurance Scheme and the Association of Specialists have the right to practise under the Health Insurance Scheme.

To begin in a practice, whether in an existing one or a new one, it is necessary to have the approval of the Health Insurance Scheme and the Association of Specialists. The system does not make any stipulations with respect to patient limitation, neither does it stipulate that any increase in the number of consultations should automatically lead to the employment of more specialists. The reason for this divergence from the norm in general practice is that agreement has not been reached on a method of regulation, partly because recourse to specialist consultations differs greatly from region to region, and partly because specialist practice is generally a supplement or alternative to hospital out-patient departments.

Committees have been established, both nationally and locally, which have an equal number of representatives of the Health Insurance Scheme and practising specialists.

2.7 Organizational Relationships

There are three doctors' negotiating organizations: one for registrars and senior registrars, one for GPs and one for specialists. The organizations negotiate independently, but the final result of negotiations must be approved by their common governing body – the Danish Medical Association – to which nearly all doctors in Denmark belong.

The counties have established a joint negotiating committee which negotiates with all employee organizations in the hospital service, including doctors' associations. A joint negotiating committee has also been established for the Health Insurance Scheme area.

The Ministry of the Interior has no direct negotiating powers concerning the labour market. In the area of the Health Insurance Scheme, however, legislation provides that the Ministry of the Interior must approve the outcome of negotiations before any agreement can come into effect. This right of approval is used in certain cases to impose conditions on the parties so that agreement can be reached.

Doctors at the top of their profession are generally in the same income bracket, in that the medical superintendent's salary is used as the basis for the regulation of salaries in general practice and specialist practice. The highest paid doctors are the practising specialists, while the lowest paid are doctors employed at the universities. Hospital registrars' salaries vary according to seniority and rank, and on the whole reflect the level for other publicly employed academics.

Danish doctors also have access to employment throughout the European Community. Of greater actual importance in connection with emigration, however, is the existence of a common Scandinavian employment market for medical personnel.

3 Sources of Information Concerning Medical Demography

Studies of the number of doctors, their main occupation and establishment conditions have been compiled at regular intervals since the beginning of the century. Figures are available to the public in the Medical Reports of the National Board of Health.

3.1 Population of Doctors

Information about medical demography is gathered and processed by public authorities and by professional organizations. Table 1 outlines the statistical analyses that have been regularly compiled since the beginning of the 1970s.

Overall Number of Doctors
The main source of information about the overall number of doctors is the medical census of the National Board of Health, which covers the total number of doctors with permanent Danish authorization. The census is conducted every second year and takes the form of a postal questionnaire sent to all doctors resident in Denmark, Greenland and the Faeroe Islands. Information about Danish doctors in the other Scandinavian countries is received from the central health authorities in those countries. Information about doctors in other countries is based on figures from the National Registration Office.

Doctors Employed in Hospitals
An annual report is made by the National Board of Health on the number of allocated and occupied medical posts in all hospital departments.

Doctors in General Practice
The Association of General Practitioners prepares an annual report on the number of practising doctors. This report contains detailed information about age and sex, patient structure, forms of practice and assistants in practice.

Unemployed Doctors
The Danish Medical Association makes an on-going report on doctors receiving umemployment benefits, categorized according to seniority and length of current period of unemployment.

Registrars' Training Conditions
The Association of Registrars holds a ballot of its members every second year concerning their training situation. The ballot is anonymous and has an 80%–85% response. Since 1982 the National Board of Health census has also contained information about registrars' training. The degree of concordance between the various censuses is generally very high. For medical superintendents, practising specialists and GPs it is nearly 100%, and any differences are due to varying census items and minor variations in the classification of the individual categories of doctors. For registrars and senior registrars there is a tendency to underestimate professional inactivity during periods of unemployment, with the result that the number in employment is overestimated. The deviation is 2%–3%.

Table 1. Regular sources of information about medical demography in Denmark

	Total no. of doctors	Hospitalemployed doctors	General practitioners	Practising specialists	Unemployed doctors	Training of registrars
Authority/organization	National Board of Health	National Board of Health	Association of General Practitioners	Health Insurance Scheme	Doctors' Unemployment Fund	Association of Registrars
Method of assessment	Questionaire + administrative register	Questionaire	Questionaire + administrative register	Administrative register	Administrative register	Anonymous questionaire
Degree of coverage	99%–100%	100%	99%–100%	100%	100% of those ensured	80%–85%
Census of frequency	Biennial	Annual	Annual	Annual	Monthly	Biennial
Source of puplication	Danish Medical Journal	Hospital statistics from the National Board of Health	Danish Medical Journal	Statistics from the Health Insurance Scheme	Danish Medical Journal	Danish Medical Journal
Most important information categories:						
Sex, age	+		+			
Seniority	+				+	+
Training background	+					+
Authorizations	+					+
Main occupation						
Typo of oooupation	+	+	+	+		+
Rank		+				+
Speciality	+	+		+		+
Geography	+	+	+	+	+	
Secondary occupation	+		+			
Professionally inactive	+				+	+
Abroad	+					
Special applicability	Information on all doctors	Increase in staff quotient; vacant posts	Practice practiculars	Full- and part-time	Rate in the junior employment market	Registrars' training requests

3.2 Forecasts

Forecasts of the number of doctors are compiled by both the National Board of Health and the Danish Association. The study is co-ordinated by a forecasting group in the National Board of Health in which all authorities and organizations who use medical forecasts are represented. The calculations for the forecasts are uniform, and new forecasts are made annually. However, a regular publication is not yet available.

4 Medical Demography

4.1 Development 1960–1982

In the period 1960–1982, the number of doctors with permanent Danish authorization increased from approximately 6500 to almost 16 000 (Table 2). The number of professionally active doctors in Denmark more than doubled in the same period, rising from 5500 to 12 000.

Of all professionally active doctors the number of those employed in the hospital service increased the most, and this increase was steady throughout the period. The general practice and specialist practice sectors first showed an increase in the 1970s. The classification "Others" in Table 2, which includes doctors employed at universities, in the social services and in administration, had the more substantial increase in the first half of the period 1960–1982.

An increasing number of doctors are employed abroad, primarily in neighbouring Sweden and Norway. The total number of doctors who are professionally inactive owing to retirement, unemployment or other reasons has risen. Quantitatively, this increase was most significant during the 1970s. The percentage of the total number of doctors professionally active in Denmark fell from 85% in 1960 to 76% in 1982.

Table 3 shows the development in the total number of professionally active doctors in relationship to population figures during the period 1960–1982. When the two sets of

Table 2. Number of doctors according to main occupation, 1960–1982

	No. of doctors				% distribution		% increase
	1960	1970	1980	1982	1960	1982	1960–1982
Hospitals service	2 550	3 625	6 575	6 500	39	47	294
General practice	2 100	2 100	2 875	2 900	32	18	38
Specialist practice	350	375	700	725	6	5	107
Others	525	825	1 000	1 000	8	6	90
Total professionally doctors active in Denmark	5 525	6 925	11 150	12 125	85	76	119
Professionally inactive	425	850	1 800	2 000	7	13	371
Outside Denmark	525	800	1 800	1 825	8	11	248
Total	6 475	8 575	14 750	15 950	100	100	146

Table 3. Number of inhabitants per professionally active doctor, 1960–1982

	Inhabitants per doctor				Increase as %
	1960	1970	1980	1982	1960–1982
Inhabitants per hospital doctor	1790	1355	780	685	161
Inhabitants per general practitioner	2175	2335	1780	1765	23
Inhabitants per professionally active doctor	825	710	460	420	96
Inhabitants 65+ per professionally active doctor	87	86	66	62	55

figures are compaired, the growth in the number of professionally active doctors is somewhat less than that shown in Table 2, since the population figure in the first half of the period rose by 15%. The increase in the number of doctors in relation to the elderly population has been only half that of the increase in relation to the total population. However, there has been a substantial development in the number of professionally active doctors.

The increase in the number of doctors reflects a solid growth in the number of qualified doctors graduating from medical schools (Table 4). Thus, around the annual number of new graduates rose within a couple of years from approximately 300 to over 600. The peak was reached in 1974, with 830 newly qualified doctors (accounting for about 1% of that birth cohort). The percentage of female graduates has been increasing since the middle of the 1970s and during the 1980 will account for 50% of the total number of new doctors.

4.2 Main Occupation, Sex and Age

Table 5 gives a detailed outline of the distribution of doctors within the medical profession for 1982. The distribution of doctors 10 years previously is shown for comparison. Sixty per cent of professionally active doctors were employed in the hospital service, mainly in regional and central hospitals, while 25% were in general practice and the remaining 15% were either full-time practising specialists or employed in school medical services, social services, administration and universities. Table 6 shows the distribution of full-time practising specialists in the different specialities, five of which accounted for 70%.

Table 4. Average annual medical graduate figure, 1960–1984

	Average number of new doctors per year	% women
1960–1964	225	18
1965–1969	305	19
1970–1974	665	20
1975–1979	685	26
1980–1984	710	33

Table 5. Distribution of doctors according to main occupation, 1982 and 1972

	1982 Doctors (No.)	Distribution (%)	1972 Doctors (No.)	Distribution (%)	Increase (%) 1972–1982
Hospital service	7 489	61.8	4 513	55.6	65.9
Regional hospitals	3 071	25.3	1 744	21.5	76.1
Central hospitals	2 322	19.2	1 3.01	16.1	78.5
Local hospitals	1 553	12.8	972	12.0	60.0
Psychiatric hospitals	386	3.2	324	4.0	19.1
General practice	2 901	23.9	2 183	26.9	32.9
Specialist practice	737	6.1	414	5.1	78.0
Other health servies	298	2.5	262	3.2	13.7
Social services	521	4.3	436	5.4	19.5
Universities and research	96	0.8	251	3.1	61.8
Others	78	0.6	56	0.7	39.3
Total of professionally active doctors in Denmark	12 120	100.0	8 114	100.0	49.4
Professionally inactive	1 995		962		107.4
Outside Denmark	1 833		841		118.0
Total	15 948		9 917		60.8

Table 6. Distribution of full-time practising specialists according to speciality

	Full-time practising specialitsts
Otorhinolaryngology	161
Ophthalmology	111
Psychiatry	98
Dermatology and venerology	86
Gynaecology and obstetrics	69
Other specialities	212
Total	737

Compared with the situation in 1972, there has been an increase in the number of professionally active doctors in all sectors except the social services. It is worth noting that although the number of general practitioners has increased by one-third, their proportion in the total number of doctors has been reduced because the number of hospital doctors and practising specialists have increased to an even greater extent. The reduction in employment within the social services is due inter alia to the transfer of duties to general practice and hospitals.

Tables 7 and 8, together with Figs. 2, 3 und 4, show the distribution of doctors according to age, sex and main occupation. Table 7 und Fig. 1 reveal that 50% of the total number of doctors are under 40 years of age. Furthermore, it appears that the proportion of women doctors is steadily rising, and ranges from one-sixth amongst the oldest to one-third amongst the youngest.

Table 7. Classification of doctors according to age and sex, 1982

	Doctors (no.)	(%)	Women in age group (%)
–29 years	1 295	8.1	31.8
30–39 years	6 566	41.2	24.1
40–49 years	3 245	20.3	19.3
50–59 years	2 193	13.8	18.7
60–69 years	1 618	10.1	18.1
70+ years	1 031	6.5	16.0
Total	15 948	100.0	21.9

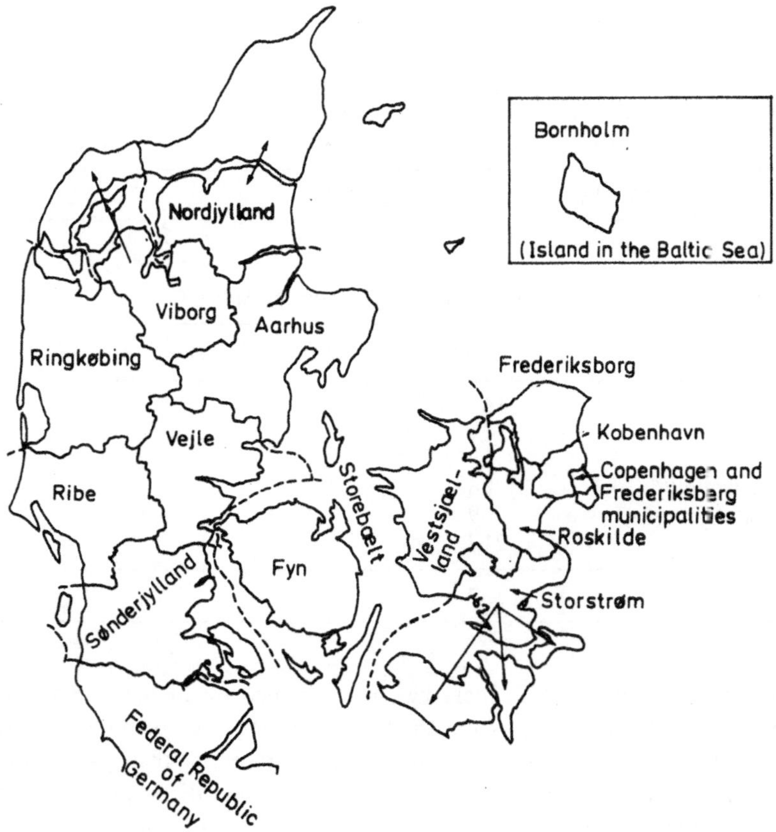

Fig. 1. The counties of Denmark

Table 8. Proportion of women in main occupation categories, 1982

	Women (%)
Hospital service	24.2
General practice	12.3
Specialist practice	27.4
Others	25.7
Total professionally active doctors in Denmark	21.7
Professionally inactive	26.2
Outside Denmark	18.2
Total	21.9

Figure 3 shows the relative distribution of the sexes in the various age groups according to main occupation. The proportion of professionally inactive doctors is somewhat larger among female doctors than among male doctors. Up until the age of 50, however, this difference is offset by a higher emigration rate among male doctors, so that the proportions of the total number of doctors who are professionally active in Denmark are almost identical for the two sexes. The proportion of females is smallest in general practice, although

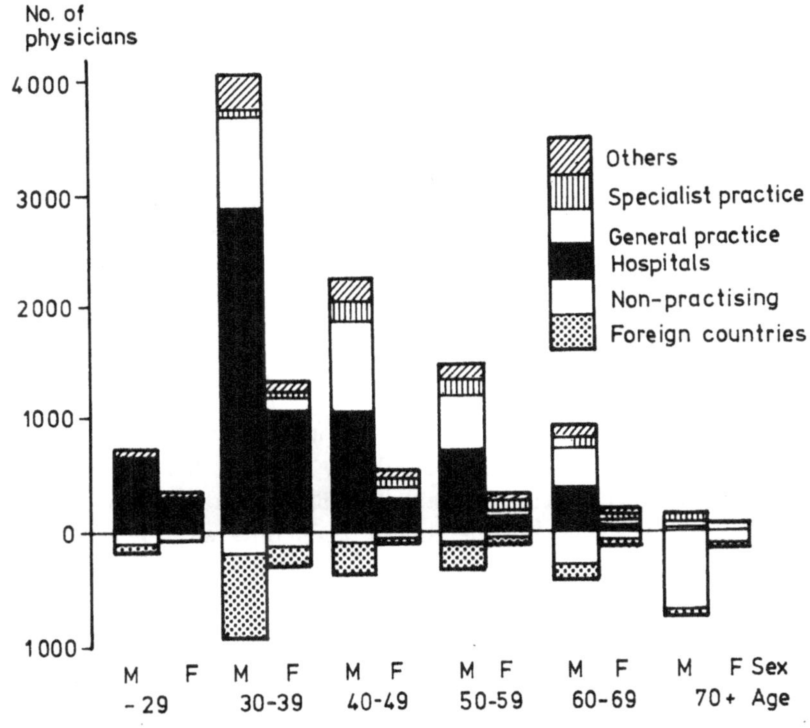

Fig. 2. Total number of doctors according to age, sex and main occupation, 1982

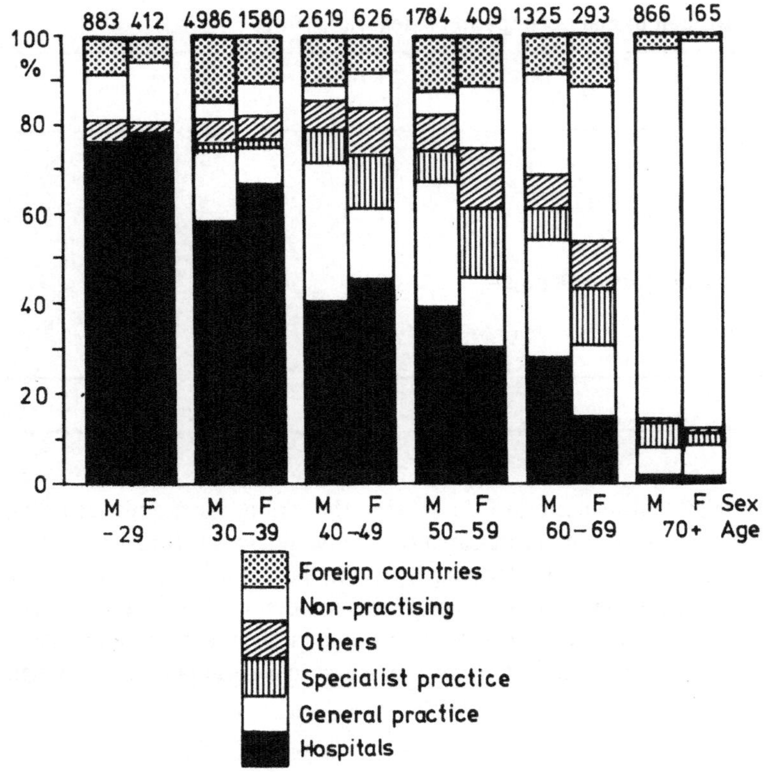

Fig. 3. Relative distribution of total number of doctors in different age groups according to main occupation, 1982

the proportion of women in executive positions such as medical superintendents in hospitals is also quite low. In particular, there are very few female superintendents in the regional hospitals.

4.3 Geographical Distribution

The ratio of professionally active doctors ranges from 1 doctor per 200 inhabitants in the central parts of the capital area to 1 doctor per 600–700 inhabitants in some counties in the western part of Denmark (Table 9). This uneven distribution reflects the location of the regional hospitals and the concentration of a range of administrative and research facilities in the capital area and in the university towns outside Copenhagen. Generally speaking, the concentration of doctors is somewhat higher in the eastern part of Denmark than in the western part. GPs are relatively evenly distributed throughout the country.

Table 10 shows how the increase in the total number of doctors during the period 1972–1982 was distributed in four main geographical regions. The relative increase in the number of doctors was greatest in the university areas outside Copenhagen, but all in all,

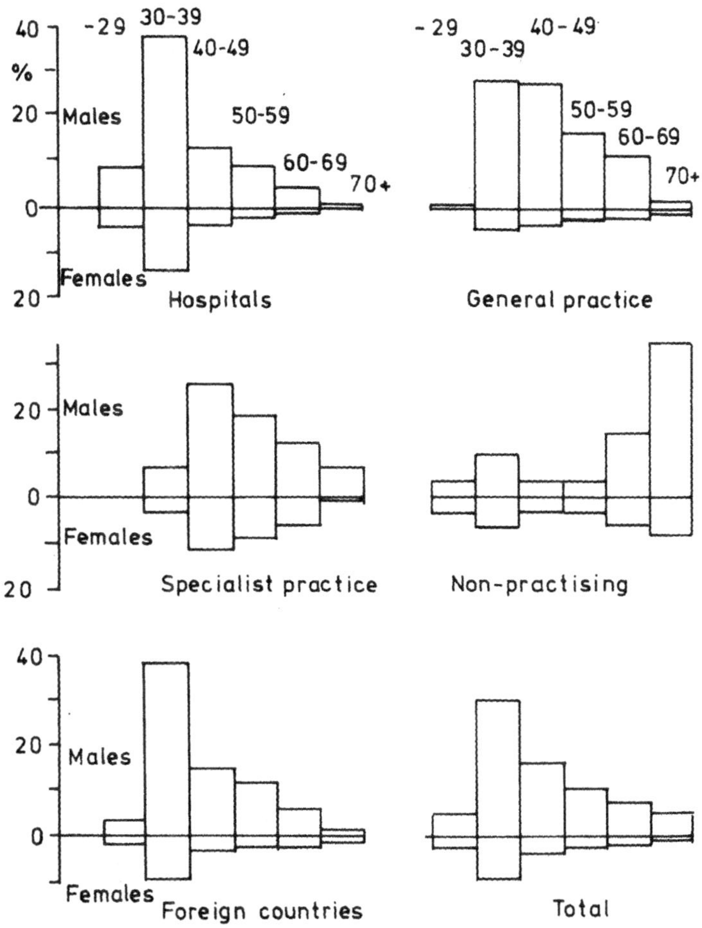

Fig. 4. Relative age and sex distribution in different sectors of main occupation, 1982

both in general practice and in the hospital service the increase has been markedly similar in the four main regions.

4.4 Specialist Authorizations

Table 11 shows the number of specialist authorizations among professionally active doctors in 1982, distributed according to speciality. The 1972 figures are shown for comparision. The actual number of specialists is somewhat lower than the number of specialist authorizations, as a number of specialists, particularly in the fields of internal medicine and surgery, have more than one specialist authorization.

Table 12 shows the distribution of specialists according to main occupation. Seventy-five per cent of specialists are employed in the hospital service, where the majority are

Table 9. Distribution of professionally active doctors in the counties, 1982

	No. of doctors				Inhabitants per doctor		
	Hospitals	General practice	Other	Total	Hospitals	General practice	Total
Eastern Denmark	4087	1310	1073	6470	568	1771	359
Capital area	3346	969	977	5292	519	1791	328
Copenhagen and Frederiksborg municipalities	1868	338	643	2820	310	1876	205
Copenhagen county	902	342	218	1491	690	1658	418
Frederiksborg county	392	183	82	657	842	1803	502
Roskilde	184	106	34	324	1109	1925	630
Vestsjaelland	382	159	44	585	728	1748	475
Storstrøm	313	149	46	508	831	1745	512
Bornholm	46	33	6	85	1022	1424	553
Western Denmark	3402	1591	657	5550	823	1758	504
Fyn	674	266	129	1069	674	1707	425
Sønderjylland	207	141	36	384	1208	1773	651
Ribe	194	118	40	352	1103	1814	608
Vejle	388	182	56	626	843	1797	522
Ringkøbing	216	144	24	384	1222	1833	688
Aarhus	914	327	264	1505	631	1765	383
Viborg	257	134	30	421	899	1724	549
Nordjylland	552	279	78	909	873	1728	530
Total	7489	2901	1730	12120	684	1765	422

Table 10. Distribution of professionally active doctors in four main regions, 1972 and 1982

	Hospital doctors per 10 000 inhabitants		Increase as %	GPs per 10 000 inhabitants		Increase as %	Total of professionally active doctors per 10 000 inhabitants		Increase as %
	1972	1982		1972	1982		1972	1982	
Capital area	12.1	19.3	60	4.2	5.6	33	21.1	30.5	45
Provinces of Eastern Denmark	7.6	12.7	67	4.8	5.9	21	13.8	20.1	47
Fyn and Aarhus counties	9.5	15.4	62	4.5	5.8	29	16.8	25.0	50
Provinces of Western Denmark	6.0	10.3	72	4.4	5.6	27	11.8	16.8	42
Total	9.1	14.6	60	4.4	5.7	30	16.3	23.7	45

Table 11. Number of certified specialists amongst professionally active doctors, 1982 and 1972

Speciality	Certified specialists	
	1982	1972
Surgery	469	407
Surgical gastro-enterology	79	49
Urology	43	17
Plastic surgery	30	17
Thoracic surgery	34	24
Orthopaedic surgery	171	94
Gynaecology and obstetrics	275	167
Neurosurgery	45	22
Otorhinolaryngology	282	204
Ophthalmology	185	129
Anaesthetics	251	164
Internal medicine	517	419
Cardiology	63	21
Pulmonary medicine	46	53
Nephrology	41	19
Gastro-enterology	44	–
Tropical diseases	12	6
Rheumatology	146	101
Long-term care	38	–
Neurology	132	116
Dermatology and venereology	133	79
Therapeutic radiology	47	23
Paediatrics	168	95
Diagnostic radiology	241	203
Pathology	133	90
Clinical serology	29	20
Clinical physiology	47	96
Clinical chemistry	96	95
Clinical microbiology	35	27
Clinical neurophysiology	15	8
Child psychiatry	62	42
Psychiatry	420	304
Total	4329	3046

medical superintendents, although a substantial number are also employed in registrar and senior registrar positions in hospitals.

The geographical distribution of specialists reflects the distribution of hospital capacity. Consequently, the number of part-time practising specialists is higher in Copenhagen and the larger towns than in the rest of the country. The geographical distribution of full-time specialists is more even.

Table 12. Distribution of professionally active specialists according to main occupation, 1982

	Specialists (no.)	%
Hospital service	2709	27.4
Medical superintendents	1783	47.6
Registrars and senior registrars	1783	24.7
Specialist practice	737	19.7
Others	294	7.9

Table 13. Professionally active doctors' secondary occupations, 1982

	Secondary occupations (no.)
Hospital service	278
General practice	561
Specialist practice	1124
Other health service	254
Training, research	360
Social sector	821
Others	226
Total	2613

4.5 Secondary Occupations

Table 13 shows doctors' secondary occupations distributed in the same categories as the main occupations. It reveals that every fourth doctor has a secondary occupation.

The greatest number of secondary occupations are to be found in specialist practice, most frequently amongst medical superintendents in the hospital service. Doctors with secondary occupations in general practice are young hospital doctors who take over GPs' duties at night and at the weekend. Secondary occupations within the social service include working as supervisory doctors for nursing homes and as advisors in the municipal social administrations. Other health services include the school health service and the industrial health service.

The total number of secondary occupations has been constant since registration started in 1976. No figures are available for the total number of hours devoted to secondary occupations, but it is generally estimated that the figure for each doctor is 5–10 hours per week.

4.6 Professionally Inactive Doctors

Of the approximately 2000 professionally inactive doctors in Denmark in 1982, about 1200 were retired. Eighty-five per cent of the latter were aged over 70 (Table 14). The

Table 14. Distribution of professionally inactive doctors according to age and reasons for absence from profession, 1982

	–39 years	40–69 years	70+ years	Total
Doctors in Denmark in age group (%)	6.7	10.7	86.1	14.1
Military service	81	0	0	81
Sick leave	63	72	0	135
Unemployment	102	26	0	128
Retirement	6	311	860	1177
Other reasons for professional inactivity	205	261	0	527
Total	457	670	860	1987

proportion of professionally inactive doctors under the age of 40 constituted 7% of the total number of doctors in that age group in Denmark. Absence from the employment market was due to military service and maternity leave only to a minor extent. The two major causes were unemployment and "professional inactivity due to other reasons". Some actual unemployment is probably concealed in the latter category.

4.7 Doctors Outside Denmark

Twelve per cent of the total number of Danish doctors authorized to practise were resident outside Denmark in 1982 (Table 15). More than 80% of them were employed within the Scandinavian-language area in the common medical employment market. Sweden was the main country for residence in the case of more than 50% of all Danish doctors employed outside Denmark. Fifty-four per cent of doctors employed abroad were under the age of 40.

The number of foreign doctors in Denmark represents only a small percentage of the total number of professionally active doctors in Denmark. Such doctors have most often come to this country for family reasons or are refugees. There are also a number of Norwegian citizens with Danish medical qualifications resident in Denmark.

5 Problems and Solutions

5.1 From a Shortage to a Surplus of Doctors

During the rapid expansion of the health service from the mid-1950s to the mid-1970s there was a constant shortage of doctors. As a consequence of the increasing number of new graduates from the medical schools from the beginning of the 1970s and the increasingly tight control of health budgets, the situation changed from one of shortage of doctors to one of surplus. At the beginning of the 1970s there was a constant 10% vacancy figure in all medical positions in the hospital service despite a strict rationing of positions

Table 15. Doctors abroad according to country of residence, 1982

	Doctors (no.)	%
Scandinavian countries	1473	80.4
Sweden	1008	55.4
Norway	301	16.4
Faeroe Islands and Greenland	127	6.9
EEC countries	128	7.0
Federal Republik of Germany	65	3.5
United Kingdom	37	2.0
United States	118	6.4
Other countries	114	6.2
Total	1833	100.0

with regard to geographical distribution. Within a couple of years the number of vacancies fell to 1%–2%, and with one exception in 1982–1983 (see below) vacancies have remained at this low level.

Even though a shortage has become a surplus, there was a rather substantial growth in the number of professionally active doctors in Denmark during the previous decade. As such, the total number of employed doctors increased by 5000, or 50%, between 1972 and 1982. One-fourth of this increase is directly due to the conversion of overtime into new registrar positions, but even when this fact is taken into account, it must be stated that there has been a considerable actual growth in the number of employed doctors.

5.2 Activity in the Health Service and Demand for Doctors

To what extent the growth in the number of employed doctors corresponds to a rising need for medical care in the population or is caused by a general increase in welfare and a greater supply of doctors is not apparent. The infant mortality rate is constantly falling, whilst the average life expectancy has remained unchanged since the 1960s, although the life expectancy for older women is still rising. The most noticeable phenomenon during the recent decade has been the growing proportion of elderly people, and particularly the increase in the number of people over 80 years of age.

Tables 16 and 17 give some figures for the increased activity in general practice and in the hospital service, respectively, during the last decade.

In general practice, there was an almost parallel growth in the number of consultations and the number of doctors. In specialist practice, there was a corresponding development, but the increase in the number of consultations and the number of doctors was higher than in general practice.

The number of doctors in the hospital service increased considerably more than the number of admittances and out-patient treatments. Sub-specialization was carried on during the period, and the elderly formed a growing proportion of hospital patients. Part of the increase in the number of doctors was due to the conversion of overtime amongst registrars

Table 16. Number of consultations in general practice, 1973–1982 (in millions)

	Consultations (no.)			Increase (%)
	1973	1977	1982	1973–1982
Category 1 patients	15.4	19.3	22.2	45
Category 2 patients	1.2	0.9	0.7	–44
Total	16.6	20.3	22.9	38

Table 17. Capacity, activity and personnel resources in the hospital service, 1972–1982

	1972	1977	1982	Increase as % 1972–1982
Capacity				
No. of hospitals	137	136	127	– 7.3
No. of beds	42 400	43 800	40 400	– 4.7
Activity				
Total admissions	820 000	927 000	957 000	16.7
Somatic admissions 0–14 years	139 000	162 700	153 300	10.1
Somatic admissions 15–69 years	526 100	580 900	582 100	10.6
Somatic admissions 70+ years	112 400	143 200	172 900	53.8
Total bed days	13.2 million	12.8 million	11.4 million	–13.6
Average length of stay (in days)	11.8	10.4	9.2	–22.0
No. of out-patient visits	2.8 million[a]	3.1 million	3.4 million	21.4
Personnel resources				
Recalculated full-time employed total	73 000	82 500	90 700	24.2
No. of doctors	4 800	5 800	7 200	50.0

[a] 1975 figure.

and senior registrars. The doctors allocated to the hospitals were new graduates from the universities.

Table 18 shows sex- and age-adjusted index figures for costs in general practice, specialist practice and the hospital service in the counties. Costs for general practice are relatively uniformly distributed, corresponding to the relatively even distribution of GPs throughout the country. Costs for specialist services and hospital treatment are, on the contrary, very irregularly distributed and are by far the highest in the capital area, where there is also the greatest supply of specialized medical care.

Table 18. Sex- and age-adjusted index figures for costs per county in general practice, specialist practice and hospital service per inhabitant, 1982

	General practice	Specialist practice	Hospital service
Copenhagen and Frederiksborg municipalities	95	148	137
Copenhagen county	102	149	101
Frederiksborg	101	150	99
Roskilde	113	125	111
Vestsjaelland	99	78	98
Storstrøm	97	85	81
Bornholm	106	43	88
Fyn	102	86	88
Sønderjylland	102	86	88
Ribe	103	72	85
Vejle	97	76	85
Ringkøbing	105	58	85
Aarhus	99	87	104
Viborg	100	74	96
Nordjylland	98	65	90
Whole country	100	100	100

Whole county = index 100.

The use of specialist services varies with the availability of specialists and the income of the population, the higher income levels making greater use of specialist services. Use of hospital facilities varies in a more complex fashion and is related to both need and supply factors. Use is highest in areas with high mortality, and many single and low incomes. Even when these factors are taken into account, it is also clear, however, that the availability of hospitals has an influence on the extent of their utilization.

Real growth in health service costs was 5%–6% a year in the early 1970s, but in the latter part of the 1970s and at the beginning of the 1980s fell to approximately 1% a year. A number of measures have been taken to limit the growth in health care costs, including various interventions aimed at limiting the supply of doctors. Furthermore, there has been a conversion of overtime amongst hospital registrars in order to distribute existing medical work to more doctors.

5.3 Restricted Entry into Medical Schools

By the end of the 1960s it was already clear that the supply of doctors would rise rapidly during the following decade. Serious discussions began in 1971 after the publication of the first actual supply forecast, which showed that the number of doctors would triple within 25 years in access to medical study continued at the same rate.

Restricted entry into medical school could not be introduced immediately, partly because there was a shortage of doctors at the time the problem was raised, and partly because many feared that restriction would lead to further social inequality in the recruitment of doctors. Finally, unemployment, especially among young people, was on the increase. Even though unemployment was predicted in the medical profession, it was small in relation to the forecasts for other professions with extended university training.

The *numerus clausus* was eventually introduced in a limited form in 1976. As a result, the annual number of new medical school graduates was reduced from just over 700 to 600. The health authorities, i.e. the Ministry of the Interior and the County Councils, had wanted the number of new doctors reducted to 450 a year. The *numerus clausus* was tightened in 1981, 1984 and 1985. With the latest reductions, the number of new doctors a year in the first half of the 1990s will be down to approximately 400 (Fig. 5). In the long term, this corresponds to the annual number of new doctors necessary to keep the present total balanced.

Altogether, the process will have taken more than 20 years, from the recognition of the problem at the end of the 1960s to the full effect of limitation at the beginning of the 1990s. Since the limitation will result in cut-backs in the universities in the coming years, it is difficult to predict how the previous research potential can be kept intact.

5.4 Regulation of Practices

In the early 1970s recruitment to general practice rose markedly, that sector having been fairly constant for decades. Whilst the hospital service expanded rapidly in the 1960s, there was a decrease in the number of practitioners in relation to the total population. In view of the large number of new doctors, the lack of good training positions in the hospital service and an increasing concern for primary care, many newly qualified doctors set up in general practice. The requirement for authorization as a GP in the early 1970s was only two years' hospital training, and it was therefore possible to sep up in general practice only a few years after graduation from medical school.

The number of consultations in general practice rose rapidly, in keeping with the arrival of more practitioners, and the Health Insurance Scheme desired some form of regulation of the profession. Similarly, once the immediate pressure of work had been relieved, doctors were also interested in regulation, since too large an influx into the profession would threaten the economic foundation of their practice.

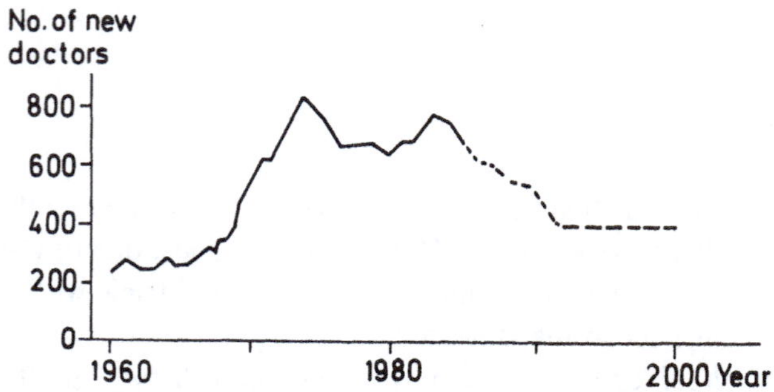

Fig. 5. Annual number of new doctors, 1960–2000

The result was a regulatory agreement in 1976, which was described above. Since that agreement, the rise in the number of consultations and new practitioners has been substantially reduced.

It did not prove possible to introduce without conflict. The Health Insurance Scheme wanted direct regulation of the number of doctors, whilst practitioners preferred regulation which would be followed by an increase in the number of consultations, thus leading to more practitioners. This model was finally accepted, but it was clear that the health authorities were not satisfied with the "automatism" of the regulation, and a renewed conflict took place in 1984. The basic regulation method is, however, still intact.

There was also a rapid growth in the number of practising specialists during the 1970s, particularly part-time practitioners. Previously, full-time pracising specialists had been concentrated in the fields of otology and ophthalmology, but as of the mid-1970s there was a substantial increase in all specialist fields, not least in psychiatry and gynaecology. Regulation in the specialist area was introducted in 1979, but in contrast to general practice, it did not preclude the possibility that an increasing number of consultations would lead to more specialists. It is more difficult to regulate specialist practice and, in addition, it is clear that the health authorities will not accept the same conditions for its regulation as have had to be accepted for general practice. It is interesting in this connection that the number of consultations in specialist practice is increasing considerably more than in general practice. The reason for this is presumably that the demand for specialist services is not yet fully met in all fields and in all parts of the country.

5.5 Conversion of Overtime

The growth in the number of doctors throughout the 1970s and the fact that there was no longer a shortage of doctors but a surplus had a particular impact on the youngest doctors. Table 19 shows the net distribution of new doctors during the period 1972–1982 to new positions and to replacement positions resulting from death or retirement, professional inactivity or employment abroad. It also shows that proportion of new positions which were due to new allocations and to conversion of overtime, respectively.

There was a larger net emigration to Sweden and Norway at the beginning of the period, when one out of five new medical school graduates emigrated. As a result of the growth in the number of doctors in Sweden and Norway, emigration ceased and in the latter part of the period the proportion of professionally inactive doctors in Denmark rose.

In the mid-1970s, the conversion of overtime became the most important demand of hospital registrars. The maximum number of obligatory weekly working hours in hospitals was 60, and it was clear that a number of new positions could be created if overtime were discontinued.

The County Councils were willing to co-operate in the distribution of existing medical work to more doctors. It was found, however, that the conversion of overtime into new jobs should result in some savings. Furthermore, the counties wanted a thorough reorganization of working conditions for hospital registrars, including the surrender of a number of "privileges" dating from the time of the doctors shortage.

Conversion of overtime was introduced to some extent in 1979 and to a larger extent in 1982. Negotiations concerning the terms for the conversion of overtime led to a dispute

Table 19. Net distribution of new doctors, 1972–1982

	No.	%
Replacement of doctors owing to death or retirement	1400	20
New posts	4000	57
Real increase in number of employed doctors	3000	43
Conversion of overtime	1000	14
Professionally inactive doctors	600	9
Emigration	1000	14
Total	7000	100

between the parties which lasted nearly 10 years, and a solution was achieved only after considerable conflict. The final solution was an economically more detrimental one than they would have accepted at the outset. Conversely, the number of positions was much greater than expected, owing to the introduction of a strict 40-hour norm. On the whole, the conversion of overtime resulted in a net increase in expenditure for the counties, and even though the doctors later had to relax the 40-hour norm, the conversion of overtime still represents a net increase in expenditure.

Generally speaking, the conversion of overtime led to a 35% increase in the number of registrar positions in 1982–1983. This dramatic increase halted the growth in the number of professionally inactive doctors, but since 1984 position quotas have again been full and there are no substantial possibilities for new job creation with regard to hospital registrars and senior registrars.

The geographical distribution agreements on the number of medical positions were discontinued in the middle of the 1970s when the supply of doctors was sufficient to ensure medical cover in all parts of the country. The large adjustment in the number of hospital registrar positions in 1982 was implemented without rationing of positions, and this showed that there were still areas of the country which were particularly prone to a lack of doctors. Some areas in the western part of Denmark had a 25% deficit in the quota of doctors in 1982, and it was only after a new geographical distribution agreement and the arrival of new doctors from medical school that the pre-1982 situation was gradually re-established.

Despite the sudden creation of new job prospects in Denmark, only a small number of Danish doctors employed abroad have returned. One reason for this may be that Danish doctors employed abroad do not wish to interrupt their present postgraduate training. Another reason may be that those who emigrated in the 1970s have now settled permanently in Sweden and Norway and will never return. A current appraisal of the emigration of Danish doctors to the Scandinavian employment market points to the fact that doctors who have remained abroad for over 4 or 5 years have little tendency to return.

5.6 Further Training

The increase in number of doctors from the beginning of the 1970s has created a number of problems in further training. Firstly, the reversal from a shortage to a surplus of doctors has caused uncertainty with regard to further training, which has been especially noticed by younger doctors. This is reflected in sporadic substitute work, fluctuating levels of emigration, unemployment, and training posts of insignificant value.

Secondly, the number of doctors pursuing further training has risen sharply in relation to the number of doctors who have finished their training. The ratio between the number of specialists and the number of nonspecialists in the Hospital Service changed from 1 : 1 to 1 : 2 in 1982.

Thirdly, the reduction in the number of working hours per week extended the time required to develop a number of practical skills. This has given rise for concern, not least of all within the surgical sector.

Finally, the number of key positions within training are not dimensioned inasmuch as all doctors will be able to attain authorization as specialists or general practitioners. In 1982, it was calculated that every third junior doctor in hospital employment actually belonged to a 'surplus group' without the possibility of achieving a full occupational authorization.

Conversely, it is also clear that the sharpened competition among doctors in a variety of areas has given rise to an increase in the standard of qualification amongst the doctors who compete successfully.

To counter the problems in further training which the large volume of doctors has created, various initiatives towards improvement have been taken. A rota system was established at the end of the 1970s; it is 18 years in duration and ensures all doctors a common minimum basic training. The training period for both general practitioners and specialists has been extended, and training positions have been established in general practice – which has a vast unused training potential. Better control has also been established concerning the directing of specialist output in the individual fields. The lengthy dispute between the hospital registrars and the country councils concerning terms for a 40-hour week has been hindering, however, improvement of training in various areas. Since the terms for a 40-hour week have been decided, there is hope that the problems affecting further training will be solved more fundamentally. It is rather important in this connection to re-establish a reasonable balance between the number of doctors in training positions and the number of doctors who are finished with their training and are employed in regular positions.

6 Forecasts

In keeping with the endeavours made during the 1970s to achieve a better balance between doctor supply and demand, quite detailed forecasts have been produced concerning the future development of supply with regard to sex and age structure, mortality, early retirement, frequency of emigration, specialist distribution etc. On the demand side, the forecasts are more of an evaluative character, partly because a sufficiently effective method of predicting the growth of demand has not been developed and, partly because future demand ist dependent on a wide range of technological, economic, political and health factors which cannot be predicted.

An account of main trends predicted in the expansion of supply in the coming decades is given below. This is followed by a discussion of a number of supply and demand factors which will tend to bring about a better balance or a greater imbalance in the future employment market for doctors.

6.1 Supply Forecasts

Figure 6 shows how the overall number of doctors with permanent Danish authorization and the number of potentially professionally active doctors in Denmark will develop in the coming decades. The phrase "potentially active doctors" refers to all doctors under 70 who are not permanently out of the Danish employment market because they have retired, have commitments abroad or are pursuing non-medical careers. The basis for the forecast is that shown in Fig. 5, which concerns the growth in the number of graduates. The forecast is that numbers will fall to approximately 400 a year at the beginning of the 1990s and remain static.

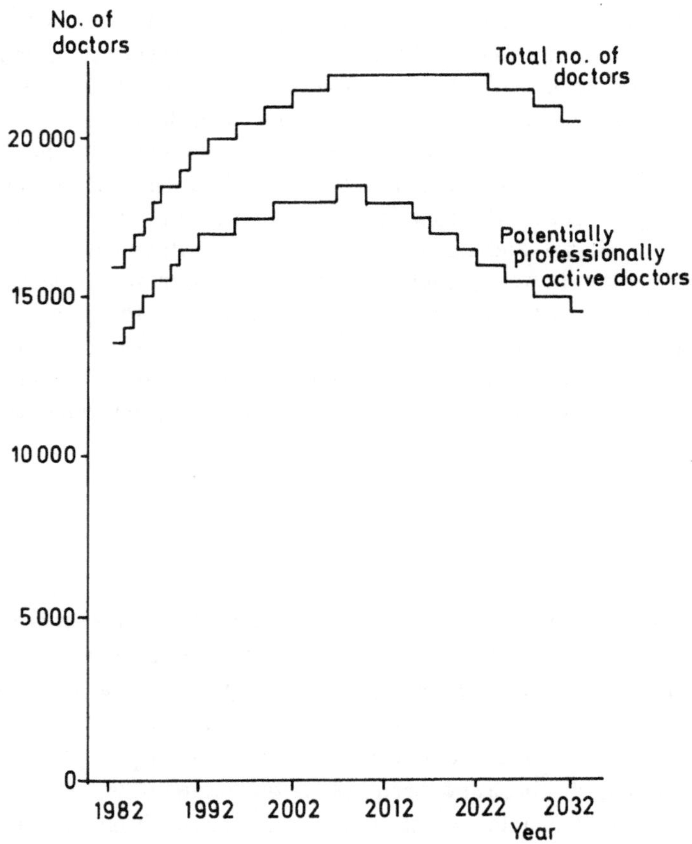

Fig. 6. Total number of doctors and numbers of potentially professionally active doctors, 1982–2032

It is assumed in Fig. 6 that there were approximately 13500 potentially active doctors in 1982, a figure which would rise to 18000 by the year 2010. The increase would be both absolute and, relatively, most rapid in the period up to the mid-1990s, since the average annual increase would be about 3%. Subsequently, the rate of increase would fall to between 1% and 1/2%, continuing towards the year 2005. As from 2010, the large number of doctors who qualified in the 1970s would begin to retire and the overall number of potentially professionally active doctors would decrease. In the long term, the figure of 400 new graduates a year would be in harmony with the present population of doctors. Figure 7 indicates that there will be a great age disparity in the population of doctors. In 1982 doctors under 40 years of age comprised 50% of the total number of professionally active doctors. This figure will fall to 25% during the next 20 years. Similarly, the proportion of middle-aged doctors will rise to nearly two-thirds of all professionally active doctors. This growth will entail problems in job structure and the distribution of duties amongst doctors.

The proportion of women is expected to comprise one-third of the total number of professionally active doctors around the turn of the century. It will be far into the next century before women comprise 50% of the total if the present sex ratio among new graduates continues.

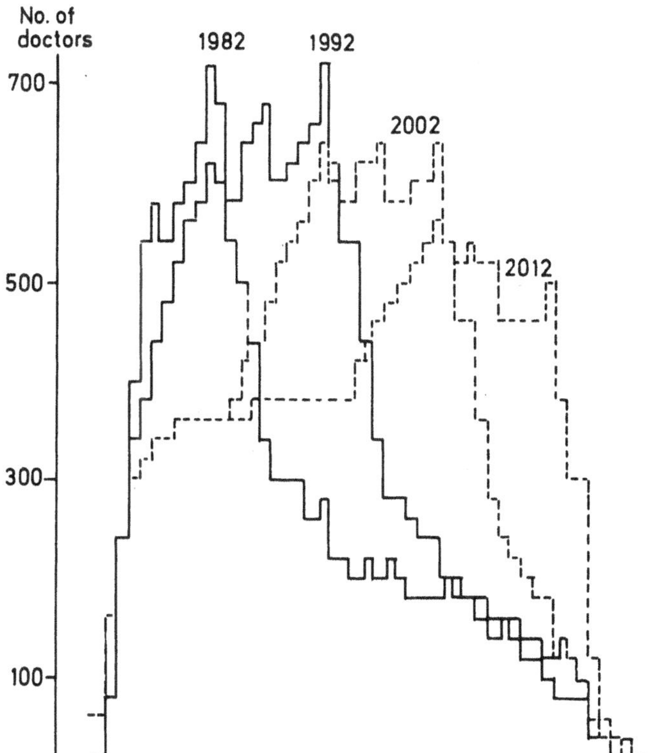

Fig. 7. Age distribution among potentially professionally active doctors, 1982–2012

6.2 Supply and Demand: Can There be an Equilibrium?

Figure 8 shows how the demand for doctors will increase in relation to the supply of potentially professionally active doctors if demand in the next 20–30 years increases on average by 0%, 1%, 2% and 3%, successively, the starting point being the actual demand in 1982.

In the long term, there will be a balance between supply and demand if demand increases between 1% and 2% a year. However, in the shorter term, i.e. within the next 10 years, it will be necessary to have a minimum increase in demand of 3% a year if there is to be a balance between supply and demand. As from the middle of the 1990s, an annual increase in demand of 1% will be sufficient to maintain the balance, and as from the beginning of the next century, there should be a balance with an annual increase of 0%. If, at that time, demand still contiues to rise, it may be necessary once again to increase the medical school intake.

It can generally be assumed that the majority of the problems in maintaining a balance between supply and demand in the future employment market will occur within the next 10 years. If the demand for doctors does not rise substantially in the coming years, or if no limitations are imposed on the supply of potentially professionally active doctors, approximately 3000 doctors will become unemployed during the next 10 years.

Table 20 gives a list of supply and demand factors which will tend in the coming years to bring about a relatively better balance or a greater imbalance in the empoyment market.

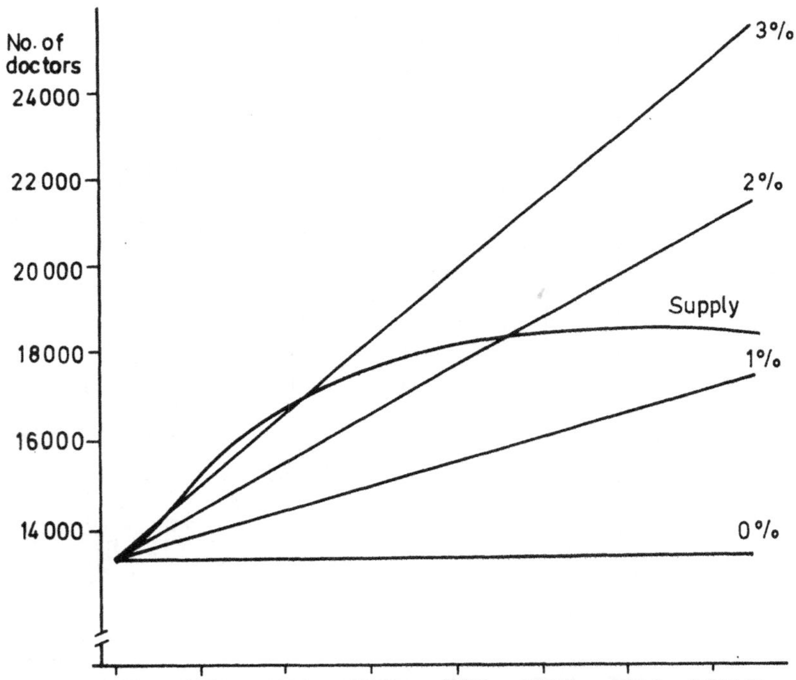

Fig. 8. Supply of potentially professionally active doctors, and alternatives for development in demand, 1982–2012

Table 20. Supply and demand factors in the medical employment market which will cause movement towards equilibrium (+) or away from equilibrium (–)

	Equilibrium
Supply	
More doctors	–
Rising average qualification standard	–
Earlier retirement	+
Reduced working hours	+
Conversion of secondary occupations into main occupations	+
Larger proportion of women	+ ?
Return of doctors from abroad	–
Demand	
Demographic development	+
Zero growth in hospital service	–
Efficiency in hospital service	+ ?
Transference to primary sector	+ ?
New areas of work, new technology	+

Since the conversion of overtime for young doctors in 1982, there have been no substantial possibilities for further expansion in the number of registrar positions. The most important step in reducing the supply of doctors will be earlier retirement, a shorter working week for all doctors and the conversion of secondary occupation to main occupation.

On the demand side, demographic development will ensure that demand will increase by 1/2%–1% a year until the turn of the century, because of the growth in the number of elderly people. The aim of the present government is, however, to reduce the growth in the public sector, including the health service, to zero. Whether or not this aim is also valid for health care is debatable, but it is a fact that increases in costs have been very low in recent years. In the hospital service, there has been a reduction in the number of employees.

It is still uncertain how improvements in the efficiency of hospital management and attempts to transfer functions from the hospitals to the primary health service will affect the employment situation for doctors. In the last 7–8 years a substantial improvement has taken place in the efficiency of hospital management, with shorter stays, increased use of out-patient treatment and greater specialization. At the same time, expansion of the hospital service has been moderate, but the proportion of highly qualified and semi-qualified personnel has risen sharply. Continued efficiency measures and limited expansion will probably be determined by a steadily rising average qualification standard for the hospital personnel. Similarly, it is conceivable that the transfer of functions from hospitals to the primary health service will increase the proportions of highly qualified and semi-qualified personnel in the health service as a whole. Greater levels of specialized care will necessiate more advisors and consultants. The increase in the doctor population in the coming decade will be so great, however, that an approximate equilibrium between supply and demand will only be maintained if there is an increase in demand, accompanied by a corresponding limitation in the supply of medical personnel.

France

Bui Dang Ha Doan

1 The Health Systems and the Physician in France

The organization of the health care system in France is based on two principles: free choice of physician by patients and generalization of sickness insurance. The costs of physician's visits, drugs, hospital stays, etc. are reimbursed to the patients by the National Sickness Fund up to 75% or more, according to circumstances. When the patient is additionally insured by other institutions, the cost of health services and goods may be negligible.

The physician provides his services to patients in different places: in his own office or in the patient's home (in case of private practice); at a public hospital; or at a health centre (previously called a "dispensary"). Most health centres were set up by local authorities or non-profit organizations, with the aim of providing outpatient care and/or preventive medicine.

When a physician has a private practice, he is paid on a fee-for-service basis, but his fees are fixed nationally by an agreement signed by the medical profession and the National Sickness Fund. When a physician works in a public hospital or a health centre, he is an employee and is paid a salary or by *vacations* (i.e. he is paid on an hourly basis). In general, physicians working full-time are paid a monthly salary, whereas part-time physicians are paid by *vacations*. A physician may have one or several places of work. In particular, he may only have a private practice or may combine his practice with hospital work and some *vacations* in a health centre. Private practices (and outpatient departments of public hospitals) are not restricted to general practice. Many specialists have initial contact with patients who come directly to their office or hospital department. This does not exclude the referral process whereby the general practitioner may refer patients to relevant specialists working in private practice or in hospitals.

The French health system appears costly to many experts, but the French public is seemingly satisfied with it. Several opinion polls conducted in recent years indicated that people wanted to keep their health system unchanged.

2 Size and Composition of the Medical Profession in the Early 1980s

2.1 Number and Ratio of Physicians

On 1st January 1983 the number of physicians registered with the Medical Council (*Ordre des Medecins*) was 140 540 (138 564 in France and 1976 abroad and in overseas territories). This number does not include doctors in the armed forces or those who are civil servants ("administrators"). These two categories are numerically small (about 3000 or 4000). Two factors make the data provided by the Medical Council Register relevant. The first is the registration with the Medical Council which is required by law before any medical practice takes place. The second is the compulsory fee that every physician has to pay annually to the Medical Council. This enables the Council to identify those who die, emigrate or retire, and to update its Register. A number of retired physicians wish to remain on the Register with a view to acting occasionally as locum tenens. Therefore, the number of active civilian physicians is somewhat smaller than the total number of registered physicians. For example, of the 138 564 physicians registered at the beginning of 1983, the estimated number of active physicians was only 129000. The latter figure corresponds to a density of 236 doctors per 100000 inhabitants (Table 1). This density was only 90 in 1955 and 150 in 1975. In 1955, actice civilian physicians numbered 39 100 and 20 years later, 78 800.

In recent decades, there has been a tremendous increase in the number and density of physicians in France. In the period 1955–1980, the number of physicians increased by 180% and their density, by 127%. Growth had been escalating since 1970. It must be emphasized that France was not in a unique position in this matter. In fact, after World

Table 1. Number and density of physicians in France (1955–1983)

January	Population (x 1000)	Physicians registered with the Medical Council[a] Active	Total	Physicians per 100 000 population
1955	43 228	39 100	39 356	90
1960	45 465	44 600	44 954	98
1965	48 687	54 300	54 764	112
1970	50 524	64 400	65 047	127
1975	52 643	78 800	81 900	150
1980	53 597	109 600	117 103	204
1983	54 546	129 000	138 564	236
1986	55 282	149 200	164 235	270

[a] Physicians in the Armed Forces and those living outside metropolitan France are not included.

War II, the medical profession in nearly all developed countries grew rapidly. For instance, in Denmark, there were 112 physicians per 100 000 inhabitants at the end of 1955, but by the end of 1978 the density had risen to 207 (Fig. 1). In the Netherlands, the two figures were 102 and 179, respectively. In Italy, there was a combined total of 138 doctors of medicine and ondotology per 100 000 inhabitants in December 1955, as against 267 in December 1978. (Data taken from the *World Health Statistics Annual* published by the World Health Organization, Geneva.) Various factors were responsible for such a universal upward trend, e.g. the tremendous increase in the size of the whole of the higher education system. As a matter of fact, the medical profession was not the only university-level group to experience a high rate of growth.

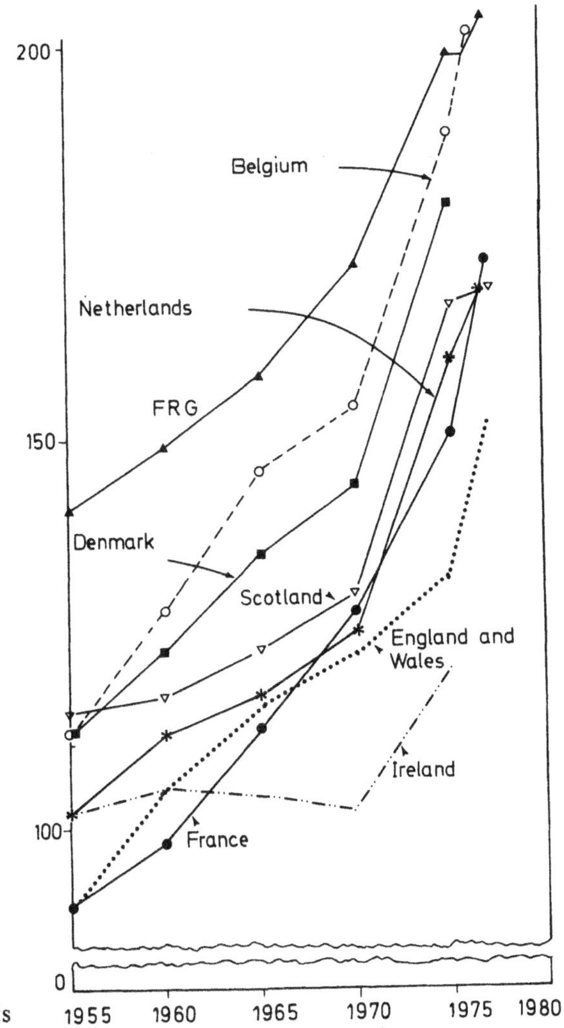

Fig. 1. Physicians per 100 000 inhabitants

2.2 Composition of the Medical Profession

The growth in the medical profession took place at the same time as many other changes in its structure or composition. First of all, let us deal with changes in its demographic structure. During these last decades, the number of female physicians increased much more rapidly than that of their male colleagues, and consequently there was a huge growth in the proportion of female physicians. In the early 1960s, female physicians totalled less than 10% of the medical profession. Twenty years later, in 1980, the proportion was 20% and in 1983, 25%. The proportion of young physicians was also growing rapidly. Physicians under 35 years old totalled less than 20% of the medical profession in 1962 but more than 37% in 1983. From the demographic viewpoint, this is easily explained by the rapid growth in the size of the profession.

Other structural changes have taken place during the past quarter of a century. Related to the institutional context of medical practice, the period 1945–1955 was a time of growth for the health centres, and a great number of medical graduates in that period therefore became full-time or part-time practitioners in these centres. The period 1960–1975 was marked by the reform of the public hospital system and the introduction into it of full-time doctors. Before 1960, doctors had only done part-time work in hospitals. As a result of these two developments and the fact that the annual number of medical graduates was stable and remained at 2200–2500, the number of young physicians setting up in private practice each year was relatively small. Since the demand for health services was soaring, it was increasingly felt that there was a shortage of physicians. It is noteworthy that such a feeling was not confined to France but was shared by a great number of Western countries, particularly during the second half of the 1960s and during the early 1970s. It disappeared after 1975, when the annual number of new medical graduates rose sharply to 7499. There were 9186 in 1977 and 8687 in 1979.

In the field of the private practice, specialist qualifications were introduced in 1947–1949. During the next two decades, new specialities were added by law to the official list and formed part of the move towards specialization. As a matter of fact, up until 1970, more and more physicians became specialists. This trend and the expansion of full-time hospital work largely halted the entry of new graduates into general practice. In other words, around 1970, the French health system was seemingly facing a shortage of physicians in general und a shortage of general practitioners in particular. Once again, it must be emphasized that many developed countries were in the same situation. As far as France was concerned, the trend was reversed after 1973–1975, when full-time hospital posts became scarce and examinations for specialist qualifications much more difficult. The number of new graduates who became general practitioners rose again after 1975.

In mid-1983, of 133 500 active physicians, 41% were general practitioners and 38% were specialists. Both categories practised in their consulting rooms as well as in public hospitals or health centres. The remaining 21% comprised those who were employed in preventive medicine or in the pharmaceutical industry, or by the National Sickness Fund in a supervisory capacity, or were not yet in practice (Table 2). The percentages in mid-1983 concerning place of work were as follows: 68% of physicians were in private practice, 30% in public hospitals, 24% in health centres or similar organizations, and 4% in other places. The total exceeds 100% since many physicians had more than one place of work. On the other hand, some of the 133 500 active physicians, particularly new graduates, were not yet working.

Table 2. Distribution of physicians in France, mid-1983

	Number	%
Total number of active physicians (July 1983)	133 543	100.0
Distribution according to place of work[a]		
Private practice	91 060	68.2
Public hospital	39 825	29.8
Health centres or similar	32 341	24.2
Other places of work	4 656	3.5
Distribution according to technical orientation		
General practice, including hospital practice	55 066	41.2
Specialities, including private practice	50 595	37.9
Other (administration, preventive medicine, not yet in practice, etc.)	27 882	20.9

[a] A physician with two places of work is counted twice.

3 Future Development

3.1 The Numerus Clausus System

Future development of the medical profession in France is closely related to the *numerus clausus* system, which was implemented in 1972. The principles of the system are: (a) students who have successfully completed their secondary school education (at the age of 17 or 18) are all entitled to enrol for the 1st year of medical training; (b) the *numerus clausus* examination takes place at the end of this 1st year; (c) the annual number of students allowed to enrol for the 2nd year of medical training is determined by the government (this number is called "legal" here).

During the first years of the *numerus clausus* system (1972–1977), the legal number of students fixed by the government was relatively high. Moreover, the effective number of students enrolled for the 2nd year of medical school was even higher, for two reasons. First, many students who did not pass the end-of-year examinations were not allowed to proceed to the 3rd year. They then repeated the 2nd year. The second reason was more important: many medical schools enrolled more students for the 2nd year of studies than the legal number.

From 1978 onwards, stricter control was enforced, and the gap resulting from the second factor was progressively reduced. The number of newly enrolled students in the 2nd year of medical training is now very close to the legal number (Fig. 2). Moreover, during the period 1978–1982 intake, both effective and legal, decreased sharply. In 1977, the number of newly enrolled students was 9171 and the legal number 8661. Five years later, the number of newly enrolled students fell to 6708 and the legal number to 6432. The legal numbers for 1983 and 1984 were even lower: 5900 and 5000, respectively. In 1986, only 4475 students were admitted into the 2nd year of medical schools.

A consensus has emerged on the need to reduce the medical school intake, and this will of course have a deep impact on the future of French medical manpower.

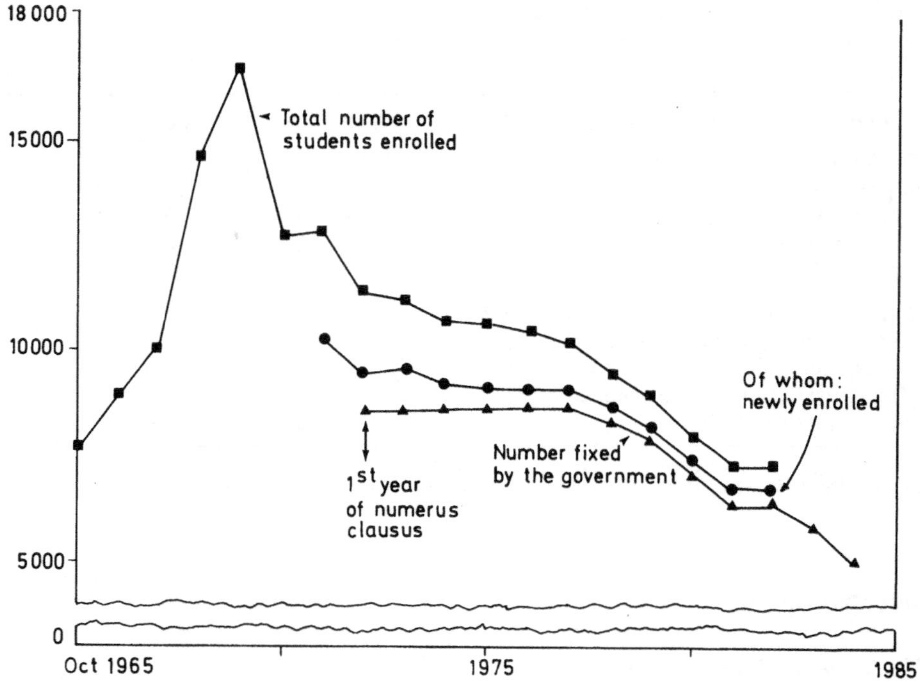

Fig. 2. Intake of medical students in France

3.2 Future Change in Size and Composition

According to a projection made in 1980, France will have 184 000 or 185 000 active physicians at the beginning of 1990, i.e. 334 or 337 doctors per 100 000 inhabitants. As mentioned above, there were 129 000 physicians 7 years earlier, in 1983. At that time, the density was 236 active physicians per 100 000 inhabitants. The projection is based on the number of students currently enrolled in medical schools and will not be affected by policies regarding future student intake. The impact of the latter will not be evident until after 1990. If the annual intake is stabilized at 5200 students, there will be 210 200 active physicians in the year 2000 and 219 900 in 2014. If the annual intake increased to 8650 students and is stabilised at this level, the medical profession will number 236 800 in the year 2000 and 288 300 in 2014. At the end of the century, the doctor density per 100 000 inhabitants will be 375 in the event of the lower student intake, and 422 in the event of the higher one.

Medical manpower will therefore continue to grow. Nevertheless, its pace will be decelerating, and the deceleration started before 1985. The medical profession will continue to grow, but increasingly more slowly. This will cause a reversal of the process mentioned earlier, and from 1983 or 1984 onwards the proportion of young physicians will decline and that of older age groups will increase. These developments will be accompanied by an increase in the proportion of female physicians. It is not impossible that by the end of the century, 35% or 40% of French physicians will be female.

None of these developments will be affected by the emigration or immigration of physicians. Up to now, medical migratory flows have not been significant, and this will probably continue to be the case, at least during the 1980s. In brief, growth in size and increase in the proportions of female and ageing physicians will constitute the three main demographic trends of medical manpower in France during the coming decades.

Though we may be able to approximate the future demographic panorama, it is much harder to forecast development in the field of professional composition. Undoubtedly, the present composition of the medical profession, by place of work or by technical orientation (see Table 2), will change; but we have no indication so far of the direction of this change. The only relevant information concerns the spacialisation of physicians: in late 1983, the planned new medical training curriculum provided for a reduction in the current annual number of newly qualified specialists (for outpatient treatment) and new hospital consultants. In other words, the bulk of future graduates will most likely become general practitioners. It is noteworthy that during the period 1975–1983, the number of general practitioners increased more rapidly than that of all French physicians combined.

4 Medical Manpower: Supply, Demand and Need

Are the present state of the medical profession and its future development relevant to an optimal provision of medical care for the population? For the time being, obviously, there is no comprehensive answer to such a question. However, some parts of it have been dealt with in France, explicitly or implicitly.

In 1970, the sixth Socal and Economic Development Plan, which covered the period 1971–1975, stated that France should have 200 active physicians per 100000 inhabitants in 1985. In early 1970, France had only 127 active physicians per 100000 inhabitants, and it was increasingly felt that there was a shortage of physicians. The objective of 200 active physicians per 100 000 inhabitants was reached in 1979, i.e. 6 years early. Meanwhile, economic slowdown, unemployment and incrasing use of health services contributed considerably to exhausting the resources of the National Sickness Fund. The order of the day was no longer to fulfil demand but to keep it under strict control.

Moreover, as a result of the generalization of sickness insurance, the regulating effect of pricing almost disappeared from the French health system, as in other Western countries. In such a situation, a greater number of physicians leads to a greater volume of medical services performed and a heavier burden on the National Sickness Fund. The need for a sharp decrease in the output of the medical training system then becomes apparent. We have seen that such an objective will not be reached significantly before 1990.

The consensus regarding the need to curb the growth of medical manpower is mainly based on economic considerations. The problem of "unnecessary provision of health services" is less frequently mentioned. It is known that certain services performed are not justified, but most people do not think that they are the main factor in the increased use of medical services. In France, as anywhere else, the various issues of over-medicalization, e.g. the negative effects of medical power, the social iatrogenic implication of modern medicine, etc., are hotly debated. Nevertheless, in general, on the Left as on the Right, it is accepted that in most cases the people's demand for health services is justified, at least partially. The problem is how to finance such a soaring demand, which is no longer regulated by market mechanisms, in a gloomy economic environment.

All this does not mean that people are naive enough to relate directly medical manpower supply to the currently available indicators of health status (e.g. life expectancy at birth, prevalence rate of diseases of various types, etc.). Indeed, it is well-known that medical manpower supply and such indicators are not closely related.

The health system and the professionals who serve in it are today at a crossroad. Expanded progressively during the three decades that followed the Second World War, the system now has to face a great number of challenges for which it was not designed. To some extent, its future success or failure will be that of all of us. The same considerations apply to the whole of the social policy system, of which the health system is a component.

Bibliography

Groupe de travail sur l'avenir du systéme de santé (1969) Reflexions sur l'avenir du systeme de santé – contribution à l'élavoration d'une politique sanitaire. La Documentation Française, Paris

Commissariat Général du Plan (1971) Rapport de la Commission Santé (série des rapports des commissions du 6ième plan: 1971–1975). La Documentation Francaise, Paris, vols 1, 2

Bui Dang Ha Doan (1973) Besoins futurs en médecins et recrutement universitaire. Centre de sociologie et de démographie médicales, Paris

Bui Dang Ha Doan (1974) Evolution numérique des médecins dans le monde (1950–1970). Rapport de statistiques sanitaires mondiales (Genève) 27 (2):84–108

Jean P (1975) Les médecins demain: pléthore ou pénurie. Cahiers de sociologie et de démographie médicales XV (1):13–15

Commissariat Général du Plan (1976) Rapport de la Commission Santé et Assurance-Maladie. La Documentation Française, Paris

Conseil Économique et Social (1979) L'adaptation des professions médicales et paramedicales aux besoins de la population française. Paris, vols 1, 2

Conseil National de l'ordre des Médecins (1980) Le corps medical et ses structures d'exercice professionnel. Bull de l'Ordre des Medecins 1:1–30

Bui Dang Ha Doan (1980) Analyse statistique de la situation des professions de santé dans le monde vers 1975. Rapport trimestriel de statistiques sanitaires mondiales (Genève) 33 (2):127–150

Federal Republic of Germany

J.F.V. Deneke

1 Structure of the Health Care System

1.1 Legal Provisions

In the Federal Republic of Germany, constitutional law prescribes that social legislation falls within the ultimate domain of the federal government. Federal legislation, in turn, determines the structure of that part of the health care system subject to social policy. However, constitutional law also specifies that the states (*Länder*) for the most part have jurisdiction over the traditional areas of governmental responsibility in the field of health. The federal government is also responsible for drafting legislation dealing with the prerequisites for taking up and pursuing the practice of medicine, whereas monitoring of the actual practice of medicine is a matter for state jurisdiction. The federal government is accordingly responsible for specifying the manner in which prospective physicians are trained (this is done in the Federal Medical Licensing Act) and for establishing the overall framework of governmental social policy within which medicine is practised. The jurisdiction of the states over regulation of the actual practice of medicine gives them governmental responsibility for ongoing medical education as well as for postgraduate training in general and specialized medicine.

The Standing Committee of the State Ministries of Health (*Ständige Konferenz der Gesundheitsminister der Länder*) helps to co-ordinate the efforts of the states and also serves to promote communication between the states and the Federal Ministry of Youth, Family Affairs and Health, as well as the Ministry of Labour and Social Affairs (which is responsible for social insurance).

Local governments and local government associations fulfil executive functions by implementing federal and state laws. The constitution also grants them sole jurisdiction over certain areas relevant to the health care system, such as their role as owner/operators of various health care facilities and their responsibility for administering public assistance (*Sozialhilfe*).

1.2 Structural Framework

The federal government, state governments and regional authorities representing local governments rely on government facilities and government public health services only to a limited extent in fulfilling their role in the health care system. Substantial and essential functions have been delegated to democratically organized autonomous administrative organs. In the realm of social welfare, the system is made more sophisticated by the involvement of institutions or entities associated by contracts to which they are common parties (*Vertragspartnerschaften*), as well as by joint facilities of public corporations performing autonomous duties, e.g. the joint administration of health insurance funds and physicians admitted to compulsory health insurance practice (*gemeinsame Selbstverwaltung der Krankenkassen und Kassenärzte*). Autonomy in the pursuit of a health profession, particularly a health profession required academic training, is exercised through professional associations with compulsory membership.

The state defines the limits of the overall framework within which private initiative is exercised in the health care system, e.g. in the areas of private health insurance; pharmaceutical production; and minimum health requirements in environmental protection, occupational health (e.g. industrial codes and trade laws) and residential hygiene.

In the light of the above, the health care system in the Federal Republic of Germany is a highly differentiated system in which market-oriented and charitable private initiatives, subsidiary autonomous activities and directives of regional authorities representing local governments are all integrated.

2 Information Relevant to Medical Demography

2.1 Data Sources

The statistical data presented in this paper and employment in its preparation were compiled from:

- Publications of the Federal Bureau of Statistics
- Publications of relevant corporations and associations involved in autonomous duties, such as the German Medical Association, the National Association of Compulsory Health Insurance Physicians, the national association of compulsory health insurance and private health insurance funds, and the national associations of pharmaceutical manufacturers
- Publications of scientific institutes, particularly the Central Research Institute of Compulsory Health Insurance Physicians in the Federal Republic of Germany, the German Hospital Research Institute, the Scientific Institute of the Association of Local

Social Health Insurance Fund and the Institute of the Professions at the Friedrich Alexander University of Erlangen-Nuremburg

In preparing the present text, preference was given to data contained in regularly collected statistics which deal with specific subjects and are collected for the express purpose of reaching conclusions about particular questions relating to those subjects. In general, great caution should be exercised when comparing bodies of data of different origin, method of collection and circumstances of compilation. This also applies to all international compendiums of health care statistics. A similar reservation is justified when examining any analysis of morbidity and mortality statistics, because motivational differences may influence the collection and processing of data, depending on the institution involved or the reason for collecting the data in the first place.

2.2 Basic Data

At the end of 1981, the Federal Bureau of Statistics found 587300 persons to be gainfully employed in health professions subject to governmental examination. Comparison of the most important professional groups in 1971 and 1981 (Table 1) reveals a 42.2% increase in the number of gainfully employed persons in this 10-year period, during which the total population increased by only 6% and the number of gainfully employed persons actually decreased by 3.7%.

The statistics of the German Medical Association show a total of 178 119 licensed physicians registered at local medical associations on 31 December 1982 in the Federal Republic of Germany, including West Berlin. Of these, 148 720 were pursuing gainful professional activities (Table 2). The average annual increase in the number of gainfully employed physicians from 1971 to the end of 1982 was 3%. As of 1982, there was one gainfully employed physician for every 415 inhabitants of the Federal Republic of Germany.

The medical employment of all physicians on 31 December 1982 was as follows:

Full-time in hospitals	41.2%
In private practice	35.0%
In civil service or public corporations	3.9%
In miscellaneous medical areas	3.3%
Not engaged in medical activities	16.5%

The trend towards an increase in the ratio between the number of physicians employed in hospitals and the number in private practice has been discernible for several years. In this regard, it should be noted that an increase in the number of newly licensed physicians „automatically" leads to disproportionately large increase in the number of physicians working in hospitals. The reason is that newly licensed doctors acquire several years' clinical experience, including postgraduate training, before they set up in private practice.

More than half of all doctors in the Federal Republic of Germany at the end of 1982 were certificated in general medicine or one of the other specialities. A substantial portion of doctors currently lacking certification are in the process of completing postgraduate training and intend to become certificated. This is illustrated by the fact that about 50% of doctors without certification are currently employed in non-supervisory posts in hospitals; a further indication is the age distribution of the group of physicians without certification (Tables 3 and 4).

Table 1. Employment levels in the health sector in 1971 and 1980

Profession	31 December 1971		31 December 1981		Change in %	
	Total	Per 10 000 inhabitants	Total	Per 10 000 inhabitants	of total (col. 3 : 1)	per 10 000 inhabitants (col. 4 : 2)
Licensed professions	166 527	272	215 330	349	+ 29.3	+ 28.3
Physicians[a]	103 910	170	142 934	232	+ 37.6	+ 36.5
Dentists[b]	31 405	51	35 501	54	+ 6.7	+ 5.9
Veterinarians[c]	8 661	14	9 441	15	+ 9.0	+ 7.1
Pharmacists[d]	22 551	37	29 454	48	+ 30.6	+ 29.7
Midwives	6 708	11	5 657	9	– 15.7	– 18.2
Non-medical health pracitioners	2 802	5	7 139	12	+ 154.8	+ 140.0
Nursing personnel[e]	172 980	282	270 673	439	+ 56.5	+ 55.7
Male and female nurses	129 342	211	200 351	325	+ 54.9	+ 54.0
Children's nurses	17 560	29	25 814	42	+ 47.0	+ 44.8
Assistant nurses	25 038	41	43 939	71	+ 75.5	+ 73.2
Maternity nurses	1 040	2	569	1	– 45.3	– 50.0
Trained pharmacy personel[f]	14 165	23	16 996	28	+ 21.7	+ 21.7
Partially licensed						
Pharmacists in training	4 604	8	–	–		
Pharmacist's assistant trainees	6 192	10	–	–		
Pharmacist's assistants	–	–	4 497	7	+ 77.8	+ 77.4
Pharmaceutical technicians	3 369	5	12 499	20		
Paramedical personnel[g]	43 128	70	61 963	100	+ 43.7	+ 42.9
Masseurs, masseuses and balneotherapists	14 319	23	21 013	34	+ 46.7	+ 47.8
Physiotherapists	6 471	11	11 485	19	+ 77.5	+ 72.7

Work and occupational therapists	873	1	3 085	5	+ 253.4	+ 400.0
Medical technicians[h]	18 998	31	22 975	37	+ 20.9	+ 19.4
Dietitians	2 467	4	3 405	6	+ 38.0	+ 50.0

[a] In 1971 there were 5445 interns.
[b] The data for 1971 include 79 officially recognized dentists.
[c] Included because of human significance; 1971 data taken from 1 July 1971, 1981 data from 31 December 1980.
[d] Data limited to those working in pharmacies.
[e] Not including nursing personnel other than that listed here, not including officially examined personnel (1971= 40 456) and not including nursing personnel in training (1971 = 51 444).
[f] Not including pharmacy aides (1971 = 26 377).
[g] Not including health inspectors and social workers (1971 = 4 586) and other persons employed in the health sector with official recognition of their occupational skills.
[h] Data from 1981 includes 5 870 radiology assistants.

Table 2. Changes in the number of physicians from 1960 to the present, broken down according to type of medical employment

Effective date	Total no. of physicians	Professionally employed physicians	Physicians gainfully employed in				
			Private practice	Hospital practice		Public authorities, public corporations, elsewhere	Physicians not engaged in medical activities
				Total	in supervisory positions		
1 January 1960	80 792	74 486	45320	21 544	4 111	7 622	6 306
1 January 1965	88 552	79 931	48 011	23 938	4 505	7 982	8 621
1 January 1970	103 981	92 773	48 830	35 066	5 860	8 877	11 208
1 January 1971	111 538	99 440	49 827	40 712	6 041	8 901	12 098
± % vs. previous year	+ 7.3	+ 7.2	+ 2.0	+ 16.1	+ 3.1	+ 0.3	+ 7.9
1 January 1972	115 977	103 470	49 897	44 110	6 197	9 463	12 507
± % vs. previous year	+ 4.0	+ 4.1	+ 0.1	+ 8.3	+ 2.6	+ 6.3	+ 3.4
1 January 1973	120 283	106 704	50 989	46 747	6 467	8 968	13 579
± % vs. previous year	+ 3.7	+ 3.1	+ 2.3	+ 6.0	+ 4.5	– 5.2	+ 8.6
1 January 1974	124 199	110 045	51 727	48 800	6 631	9 518	14 154
± % vs. previous year	+ 3.3	+ 3.1	+ 1.4	+ 4.4	+ 2.5	+ 6.1	+ 4.2
1 January 1975	130 183	114 624	52 913	51 981	7 125	9 730	15 559
± % vs. previous year	+ 4.8	+ 4.2	+ 2.3	+ 6.5	+ 7.4	+ 2.2	+ 9.9
1 January 1976	134 398	118 007	53 303	54 895	7 520	9 809	16 391
± % vs. previous year	+ 3.2	+ 3.0	+ 0.7	+ 5.6	+ 5.5	+ 0.8	+ 5.3
1 January 1977	138 895	121 500	54 974	56 616	7 686	9 910	17 395
± % vs. previous year	+ 3.3	+ 3.0	+ 3.1	+ 3.1	+ 2.2	+ 1.0	+ 6.1
1 January 1978	143 529	124 805	56 157	58 385	7 924	10 263	18 724
± % vs. previous year	+ 3.3	+ 2.7	+ 2.2	+ 3.1	+ 3.1	+ 3.6	+ 7.6

1 January 1979	150 544	129 790	57 566	62 276	8 145	9 948	20 754
± % vs. previous year	+ 4.9	+ 4.0	+ 2.5	+ 6.7	+ 2.8	– 3.1	+ 10.8
31 December 1979	158 387	135 586	58 908	65 714	8 221	10 964	22 801
± % vs. previous year	+ 5.2	+ 4.5	+ 2.3	+ 5.5	+ 0.9	+ 10.2	+ 9.9
31 December 1980	164 124	139 452	59 777	67 964	8 383	11 711	24 672
± % vs. previous year	+ 3.6	+ 2.9	+ 1.5	+ 3.4	+ 2.0	+ 6.8	+ 8.2
31 December 1981	171 569	144 224	60 652	71 724	10 047	11 848	27 345
± % vs. previous year	+ 4.5	+ 3.4	+ 1.5	+ 5.5	+ 19.8	+ 1.2	+ 10.8
31 December 1982	178 119	148 720	62 418	73 420	10 251	12 882	29 399
± % vs. previous year	+ 3.8	+ 3.1	+ 2.9	+ 2.4	+ 2.0	+ 8.7	+ 7.5

Table 3. Comprehensive overview of numbers of physicians with specialized qualifications on (Source; Statistisches Bundesamt)

	Total physicians (cols. 3+5+8+10+12)		Breakdown according to type of gainful medical employment In private practice		Total in hospitals	
	No.	Proportion per speciality	No.	Proportion of col. 1	No.	Proportion of col. 1
	Absolute	%	Absolute	%	Absolute	%
Physicians without specialized qualifications	80 850	45.4	14 183	17.5	43 540	53.9
General medicine (certificated)	17 420	9.8	13 151	75.5	556	3.2
Anesthetics	4 385	2.5	243	5.5	3 671	83.7
Occupational medicine	893	0.5	21	2.4	126	14.1
Opthalmology	3 958	2.2	2 992	75.6	429	10.8
General surgery	8 808	4.9	1 685	19.1	5 368	60.9
Dermatovenerology	2 683	1.5	1 683	62.7	379	14.1
Obstetrics and gynaecology	8 515	4.8	5 178	60.8	2 326	27.3
Otorhinolargyngology	3 317	1.9	2 248	67.8	516	15.6
Internal medicine	20 943	11.8	10 108	48.3	6 993	33.4
Paediatrics	6 647	3.7	3 122	47.0	1 830	27.5
Child psychiatry	309	0.2	73	23.6	168	54.4
Laboratory medicine	839	0.5	255	30.4	373	44.5
Respiratory medicine	1 442	0.8	362	25.1	329	22.8
Microbiology/contagous disease epidemiology	195	0.1	9	4.6	131	67.2
Maxillofacial surgery	396	0.2	168	42.4	122	30.8
Neuropsychiatry	4 594	2.6	1 752	38.1	1 926	41.9
Neurological surgery	282	0.2	17	6.0	253	89.7
Neurology	689	0.4	295	42.8	240	34.8
Nuclear medicine	220	0.1	33	15.0	175	79.5
Public health	434	0.2	1	0.2	13	3.0
Orthopaedics	3 380	1.9	2 291	67.8	700	20.7
Pathology	625	0.4	61	9.8	472	75.5
Pharmacology	300	0.2	3	1.0	158	52.7
Psychiatry	553	0.3	111	20.1	305	55.2
Radiology	3 187	1.8	1 128	35.4	1 506	47.3
Forensic medicine	127	0.1	1	0.8	79	62.2
Urology	2 128	1.2	1 244	58.5	736	34.6
Total no. of physicians	178 119	100.0	62 418	35.0	73 420	41.2

31 December 1982 (in the Federal Republic of Germany, not including Berlin)

No. in supervisory positions Absolute	With public authorities public corporations No. Absolute	Proportion of col. 1 %	In other medical activities No. Absolute	Proportion of col. 1 %	Not engaged in medical activities No. Absolute	Proportion of col. 1 %
532	3 253	4.0	3 796	4.7	16 078	19.9
57	235	1.3	236	1.4	3 242	18.6
1 213	83	1.9	68	1.6	320	7.3
25	207	23.2	427	47.8	112	12.5
102	29	0.7	61	1.5	447	11.3
1 796	223	2.5	163	1.9	1 369	15.5
85	84	3.1	63	2.3	474	17.7
882	85	1.0	76	0.9	850	10.0
148	49	1.5	27	0.8	477	14.4
2 402	997	4.8	486	2.3	2 359	11.3
435	388	5.8	118	1.8	1 189	17.9
63	30	9.7	7	2.3	31	10.0
149	73	8.7	22	2.6	116	13.8
77	193	13.4	45	3.1	513	35.6
36	37	19.0	10	5.1	8	4.1
48	8	2.0	10	2.5	88	22.2
591	235	5.1	85	1.9	596	13.0
75	5	1.8			7	2.5
86	50	7.3	5	0.7	99	14.4
73	4	1.8	4	1.8	4	1.8
3	345	79.5	11	2.5	64	14.7
228	94	2.8	27	0.8	268	7.9
197	27	4.3	9	1.4	56	9.0
46	31	10.3	63	21.0	45	15.0
53	63	11.4	8	1.4	66	11.9
604	95	3.0	55	1.7	403	12.6
17	38	29.9	6	4.7	3	2.4
288	20	0.9	13	0.6	115	5.4
10 251	6 981	3.9	5 901	3.3	29 399	16.5

Table 4. Age distribution of physicians on 31 December 1982 (in the Federal Republic of Germany, not including West Berlin)

Speciality	Total physicians		Proportion and each age group in a given speciality, expressed as % of Columny 1					
	No. Absolute	Female %	up to 34 %	35–39 %	40–49 %	50–59 %	60–65 %	66 and older %
Physicians without specialized qualifications	80 850	34.6	49.2	15.4	13.7	6.2	5.7	9.8
General medicine (certificated)	17 420	17.4	4.9	9.7	13.2	14.2	23.0	34.9
Anaesthetics	4 385	45.3	11.7	29.1	42.9	12.7	2.9	0.7
Occupational medicine	893	21.8	2.8	11.4	23.1	25.1	26.8	10.9
Opthalmology	3 958	29.3	7.1	16.1	29.8	18.2	13.3	15.4
General surgery	8 808	5.7	3.3	18.0	32.7	17.0	12.4	16.6
Dermatovenerology	2 683	34.2	5.5	13.5	28.5	13.9	16.9	21.7
Obstetrics and gynaecology	8 515	17.4	4.4	18.9	37.5	16.7	11.2	11.2
Otorhinolargyngology	3 317	11.5	5.8	14.3	27.5	17.9	14.1	20.3
Internal medicine	20 943	17.3	3.1	16.8	34.6	18.6	14.2	12.7
Paediatrics	6 647	47.5	5.0	15.3	33.5	18.8	13.5	13.9
Child psychiatry	309	50.5	3.6	23.6	40.8	15.5	10.0	6.5
Laboratory medicine	839	21.9	1.9	12.4	37.8	20.3	15.1	12.5
Respiratory medicine	1 442	25.4	1.5	5.8	11.7	11.8	29.3	39.8
Microbiology/contagous disease epidemiology	195	19.5	4.1	15.4	39.0	27.2	12.8	1.5
Maxillofacial surgery	396	3.3	7.3	21.2	29.8	17.9	6.3	17.4
Neuropsychiatry	4 594	26.8	4.0	16.4	32.6	17.1	17.4	12.6
Neurological surgery	282	4.3	2.5	23.4	45.0	19.5	6.7	2.8
Neurology	689	29.5	5.5	15.5	34.4	14.4	15.2	14.9
Nuclear medicine	220	11.4	3.6	25.0	46.4	19.1	4.1	1.8
Public health	434	34.8	3.0	10.1	25.3	22.8	30.0	8.8
Orthopaedics	3 380	7.1	4.4	21.2	36.6	16.2	12.1	9.4
Pathology	625	12.0	3.8	14.7	44.5	16.5	11.8	8.6
Pharmacology	300	12.0	1.3	10.3	36.7	24.7	15.7	11.3
Psychiatry	553	35.8	9.6	26.6	31.5	15.7	10.8	5.8
Radiology	3 187	14.3	3.1	16.7	34.5	18.5	15.8	11.4
Forensic medicine	127	14.2	2.4	15.0	37.0	25.2	18.1	2.4
Urology	2 128	1.3	3.8	20.3	45.5	14.2	10.0	6.3
Total no. of physicians	178 119	26.8	24.8	15.8	22.8	12.0	10.9	13.7

In the light of the large number of new doctors, the medical profession in the Federal Republic of Germany consists of a "young" body of physicians, about one-further of all medical active doctors being under 35 years of age. In the past 15 years, the middle-aged groups which bear the major burden of all professional responsibilities have decreased in number in comparison with the age groups comprising the young generation of doctors and the more advanced age groups in which work loads tend to be consciously reduced.

The proportion of female doctors has increased over the past decades and has now reached 27%.

Of the total number of physicians employed in the Federal Republic of Germany, including West Berlin, on 31 December 1981, 7.5% were aliens (Table 5). The regulations governing the process of admission to basic medical training reserve a certain percentage of places for foreign students. Only estimates are available, however, as to the actual number of foreign students persuing medical studies in the Federal Republic of Germany.

As in all countries, the regional distribution of physicians in the Federal Republic of Germany reveals a concentration of physicians in industrial or urban centres. Medical manpower shortages in rural and suburban areas are only temporary. The number of privately practising physicians providing out-patient medical care is steadily increasing. At the present time, there is already a surplus of applicants for medical staff positions in hospitals. Accordingly, there is a trend towards an increase both in the number of unemployed physicians actively seeking employment and in each unemployed physician's average length of unemployment.

2.3 Basic Demographic Data

2.3.1 Changes in Morbidity Statistics

Changes in population structure (age distribution and marital status) represent only one group of related data in the whole complex of influences affecting morbidity rates. Relevant basic data which do not reflect the impact of medical research or the provision of medical care includes those relating to:

- The increase in disorders resulting from environmental changes related to industrialization and from simultaneously increasing population (as this affects occupation, home, holiday, recreation)
- The increase in self-destructive behaviour resulting from consumption of alcohol, coffee, tea, cigarettes, etc., unhealthy eating habits, and hazardous and physically taxing recreational activities
- The increasing need for greater assurance of personal well-being, resulting for example from increased perception of a need for security, from increasing personal exercise of all potential legal rights to benefits, or from the influence of fashions and the media
- The increase in psycho-social conflicts, which also results, last but not least, from the above-mentioned developments
- The increasingly legal character of the doctor-patient relationship and the consequent incentive for „defensive" medicine offering services which would not necessarily be required from a strictly medical viewpoint

Table 5. Alien physicians employed in the Federal Republic of Germany on 31 December 1979 and 1981 (Source: German Medical Association Statistics)

No.	Country of origin	1979 No.	1981 No.	Change in %	Proportion of total in %
1	Belgium	78	149	+ 91.0	1.4
2	Denmark	26	38	+ 46.2	0.3
3	France	108	185	+ 71.3	1.7
4	Greece	611	653	+ 6.9	6.0
5	United Kingdom	68	93	+ 36.8	0.9
6	Ireland	4	4	± 0	–
7	Italy	128	174	+ 35.9	1.6
8	Luxembourg	75	84	+ 12.0	0.8
9	Netherlands	117	185	+ 58.1	1.7
10	Greece	1 215	1 565	+ 28.8	14.4
11	Yugoslavia	852	837	– 1.8	7.7
12	Austria	290	290	± 0	2.7
13	Poland	195	308	+ 57.9	2.8
14	Romania	235	244	+ 3.8	2.2
15	Czechoslovakia	271	302	+ 11.4	2.8
16	Turkey	1 336	1 327	– 0.7	12.2
17	Hungary	113	138	+ 22.1	1.3
18	Other countries	442	504	+ 14.0	4.6
19	Other European countries	3 734	3 950	+ 5.8	36.3
20	European total	4 949	5 515	+ 11.4	50.7
21	Egypt	121	135	+ 11.6	1.3
22	Ghana	195	164	–15.9	1.5
23	Libya	42	59	+ 40.5	0.5
24	Nigeria	88	76	–13.6	0.7
25	Other countries	207	258	+ 24.6	2.4
26	African total	653	692	+ 6.0	6.4
27	Afghanistan	105	137	+ 30.5	1.3
28	India	198	180	– 9.1	1.7
29	Indonesia	308	354	+ 14.9	3.3
30	Iraq	151	123	–18.5	1.1
31	Iran	889	879	– 1.1	8.1
32	Israel	128	166	+ 29.7	1.5
33	Jordan	268	299	+ 11.6	2.7
34	Philippines	70	99	+ 41.4	0.9
35	Syria	811	903	+ 11.3	8.3
36	Other countries	374	412	+ 10.2	3.8
37	Asian total	3 302	3 552	+ 7.6	32.7
38	North America	129	149	– 15.5	1.4
39	Central America	58	70	– 20.7	0.6
40	South America	266	306	– 15.0	2.8
41	All other countries	453	575	– 15.9	4.8
42	Physicians without nationality	8	5	–37.5	–
43	Other countries	900	590	–34.4	5.4
44	Total alien physicians	10 265	10 879	– 6.0	100.0

- The disproportionately large increase in the number of new health professions and occupations and in the total number of gainfully employed persons in the health care system, insofar as the increases are superfluous from a strictly medical viewpoint
- The expansion of medical services, even for slight health disorders, beyond the level required from a strictly medical viewpoint, concomitantly with the expansion of the concept of ill health as defined by WHO

Truly reliable information on the frequency of diseases (morbidity rates) and changes therein are not provided by existing data, which are frequently limited to specific, legally defined spheres and are thus often incomplete (e.g. hospital, health insurance fund and unemployment statistics, or cancer and myocardial infarction data banks). The most reliable sources of information today, despite inherent drawbacks, continue to be mortality rates (rates of death attributed to specific diseases). In the relevant literature, attention is called to the following development in the Federal Republic of Germany from 1952 to 1979:

- Decreasing death rates, particularly deaths from infectious and parasitic diseases (total), cancer (total), hypertension, pneumonia, ovarian cancer, gastric cancer, gastro-intestinal ulcer, inflammatory renal diseases, as well deaths caused by accidents, poisoning and silicosis
- Increasing death rates, particularly deaths from cancer of the respiratory tract, coronary artery disease (up to ca. 1970: + 85% in men, + 10% in women; subsequently, stagnation of rate in men, decrease in women), bronchitis, cirrhosis of the liver
- Stagnating death rates in respect of rheumatic diseases, diabetes, breast and prostate cancer

If diseases are grouped according to etiological factors (genetics, environmental influences, self-destructive behaviour) and the various groups compared, it will be seen that the diseases with increasing death rates are for the most part those resulting primarily from self-destructive behaviour (smoking, alcohol).

The current demographic and epidemiological changes are accompanied by a change in the spectrum of diseases. This observation applies to changes in the incidence of and death rates attributable to given diseases. It also applies, however, to the changing constellation of diseases leading to multi-morbidity. The increase in survival time has an impact on medical expenditure particularly for:

- Various cancerous diseases
- Hypertension
- Coronary or other types of heart disease
- Diabetes
- Vascular disease
- Gastro-intestinal ulcers
- Haemophilia
- Children with congenital deformities
- Leukaemia
- Renal failure
- Cystic fibrosis
- Decreasing perinatal death rate

Treatment of most chronic diseases occasionally requires lifelong application of expensive drugs (e.g. cytostatic agents, beta-blockers, anti-hypertensive agents, insulin, etc.) and/or apparatuses (cardiac pacemakers, hemodialyzers).

Realistic evaluation of various rates of morbidity and changes therein cannot be derived simply from mortality statistics. Any statistics concerning cause of death which are based on statements on death certificates pose problems, at least when "cardiovascular failure" is cited or when one is considering patients aged 50 or more in whom multi-morbidity is significant.

3 Trends

3.1 Development of the Supply of Physicians

The future development of the number of physicians per person in the Federal Republic of Germany will continue to be influenced by the number of newly licensed physicians, new admissions to basic medical training and medically employed physicians, as well as by changes in the overall population (for changes since 1960 see Figs. 1 and 2).

Future developments will be decisively influenced by the following facts:

- The increase in the number of newly licensed physicians continues clearly to exceed the birth rate, and the relative number of licensed physicians consequently increases.
- The number of physicians in private practice is increasing in the same way.
- The population total continues to stagnate, and consequently the disproportionately large increase in the number of physicians per person continues.

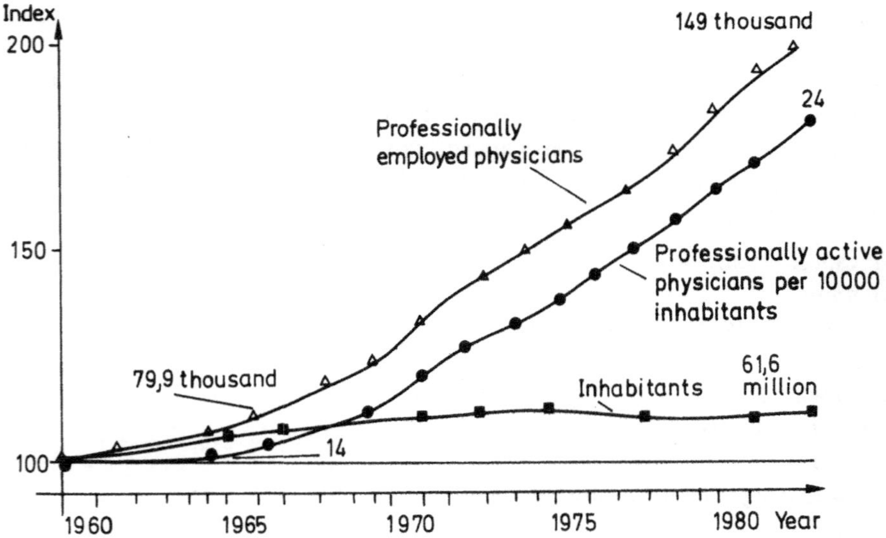

Fig. 1. Changes in the number of professionally employed physicians, the population and the number of professionally employed physicians per 10 000 inhabitants from 1960 to the present (Sources: German Medical Association and official statistics)

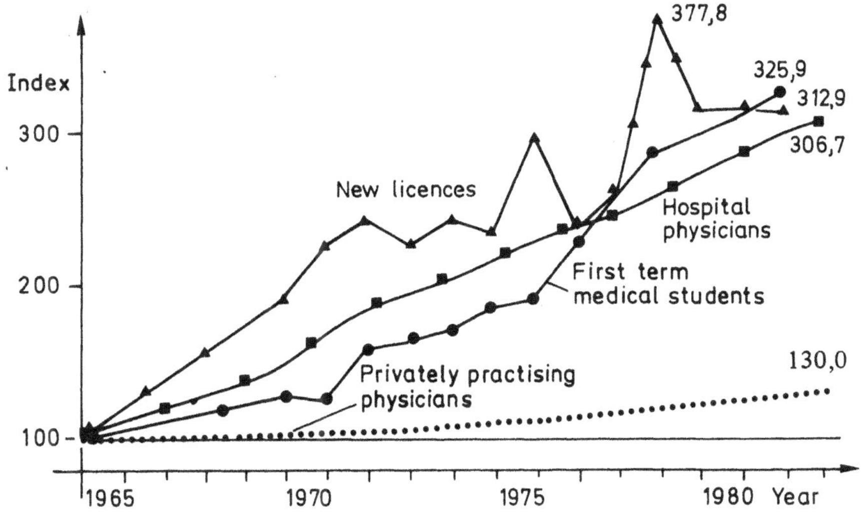

Fig. 2. Changes in the number of new licences, new medical students and physicians in private practice from 1965 to the present (Sources: German Medical Association, official statistics and author's calculations)

The difficulty in determining exactly the future need for physicians, and the diversity and interaction of factors which may influence demand were pointed out in a study by PROGNOS AG (Basel) entitled *Entwicklung des Bedarfs an Ärzten* (The development of the Demand for Physicians), which had been commissioned in 1979 by the Federal Ministry of Labour and Social Affairs, and was published in Bonn under the title of *Forschungsbericht 80* (Research Report 80) as part of a series of publications under the auspices of the Minister of Labour and Social Affairs. The following is an English translation of an excerpt from the study:

An objective, unequivocal demand for physicians does not exist. In light of the group-oriented pluralistic concept of demand on which the study is based, development of the demand for physicians rather results from the influences of involved social groups (primarily physicians, health insurance funds, citizens/patients, hospital owner/operators, the body politic and public administration, and collective wage bargaining groups) on the functional constellation of factors directly affecting the demand for physicians, including:

1. Changes in the frequency of disease (morbidity)
2. Level of service utilization and treatment volume
3. Organizational structures
4. Content and provision of services

. . . The demand for a numerical increase in the supply of physicians cannot be exactly calculated (statistical models) and reasonable estimates suggest that in the order of 20000–25 000 additional professionally active physicians will be required between 1978 and the year 2000. The demand consequently falls far short of the expected increase in the supply of physicians.

From a qualitative and structural viewpoint, there is an increasing, urgent need for physicians who are capable of effectively coping with the:

- ongoing changes in the spectrum of diseases (increase in so-called diseases of civilization induced by factors in the physical and psychosocial environment as well as individual behaviour)
- the need for economic performance in light of increasingly restricted financial leeway . . .

In closing, the PROGNOS study concluded that the future development of the demand for physicians within the framework of democratic, economic and social conditions will be decisively influenced by the behaviour of the social groups directly involved. In this regard, the study presented three possible behaviour-oriented scenarios with the following potential consequences:

Scenario I:
In the case of the previously effective domination of group egoisms continues and becomes more pronounced, the quantitative but not the qualitative aspects of the demand (for medical services) will be satisfied. Due to increasing conflicts between the need for and the capacity to provide services (as well as) expenses and financial capacity, the health care system approaches a state of collapse.

Scenario II:
Increasing governmental interference restricts the quantitative demand for physicians, while qualitative espects (of the demand) become even more severe. Although the cost and volume problems are solved, the system of medical care deteriorates as a result.

Scenario III:
Through self-regeneration of the system of self-administration accompanied by co-operative participation of all groups, a health care system results in which an equilibrium exists in terms of cost, volume and substance between the demand and supply of physicians and medical services.

Despite the *Numerus clausus* (restricted admissions policy), the number of new medical students is not strictly related to the training capacity of universities and their facilities or, to say the least, to estimates of the demand for physicians, regardless of how these may be arrived at.

In addition, the development of the health care system in the Federal Republic of Germany is characterized by the fact that the number of persons gainfully employed in non-medical health professions and occupations continues to increase more rapidly than the number of physicians, and new professional and occupational fields are being created which develop services relevant to the health care system. At the same time, the volume of self-medication is increasing progressively.

3.2 Medical Care

The system of medical care in the Federal Republic of Germany is based on a division of tasks and co-operation among the following spheres:

- Out-patient medical care
- In-patient medical care
- Public health

Table 6. Sub divisons of social insurance

Branch of insurance	Risk	Organizational pattern	Administering institutions
Compulsory unemployment insurance	Losses suffered as a result of non-self-incurred unemployment	National	Federal Institution for Labour Exchanges and Unemployment Insurance
Compulsory health insurance	Illness, impending illness, early diagnosis, treatment, disablement maternity, prevetion after-care, lump-sum death benefits	Regional	Local social health insurance funds
		Employer	Employers' health insurance funds
		Employer	Artisans' health insurance funds
		Vocational	Workmen's substitute health insurance funds
		Vocational	Salaried employees' health insurance funds
		National/vocational	Seamen's health insurance funds (Seamen's Fund)
		National/vocational	National Society of Miners
		Regional/vocational	Agricultural health insurance funds
Compulsory old-age invalidity and survivor insurance	Invalidity, old age	National/vocational	Federal Insurance Institution for salaried employees
		Regional/vocational	State insurance institutions
		National/vocational	National Society of Miners
		National/vocational (workmen)	Seamen's Fund
		National/vocational (workmen)	National Railwaymen's Insurance Institution
		Regional/vocational	Agricultural old-age funds
Workmen's compensation insurance	Occupational injury, occupational illness, death resulting from occupational injury or occupational illness	Trade/national	Artisans' workers' compensation funds
		Trade/regional	Artisans' workers' compensation funds
		Vocational/national	Agricultural workers' compensation funds
		Vocational/regional	Agricultural workers' compensation funds
		Regional	Municipal workers' compensation funds
		Regional	Cities
		Regional	State agencies
		Regional	Fire department workers' compensation funds
		National	Federal agencies
		National	Federal Institution for Labour Exchanges and Unemployment Insurance

From M. Arnold, H.-P. Brauer, J.F.V Deneke, E. Fiedler (1983) Der Beruf des Arztes in der Bundesrepublik Deutschland, 2nd edn.

Out-patient and in-patient medical care is integrated into a highly differentiated system of social security in which the compulsory and private health insurance funds play a central role (Table 6). The institutions administering compulsory health insurance (CHI) – *gesetzliche Krankenversicherung* – are the local social, employers' artisans' and farmers' health insurance funds (*Ortskrankenkassen, Betriebskrankenkassen, Innungskrankenkassen*), as well as the substitute health insurance funds (*Ersatzkrankenkassen*), the National Society of Miners and Seamen's Fund (*Bundesknappschaftkasse und Seekasse,* respectively). Compulsory health insurance covers risks of illness, pregnancy and death. Supplementary benefits include coverage of the cost of early-diagnosis examinations, maternity benefits, family assistance, lump-sum death benefits, preventive medical care and other services (for abortion or sterilization). Private health insurance (PrHI) – *private Krankenversicherung* – performs the following tasks in the overall system of social security:

- Provision of full health insurance coverage for those persons who are not legally required to be insured
- Provision of supplementary coverage for persons participating in CHI funds, in order to satisfy personal preferences exceeding CHI coverage

The number of persons with full PrHI coverage in 1982 amounted to more than 5 million. This corresponds to 8.2% of the residential population of the Federal Republic of Germany.

There was a total of 1276 individual CHI funds in the Federal Republic of Germany in December 1982. Each fund has its own history: some were established to serve a particular municipality, and others to serve certain regions, professions, occupations or groups thereof, or even individual firms. This multifarious organizational framework enabled various insurance institutions independently to shape their social health insurance protection to meet the special needs and desires of their clientele. Coverage is provided for members of a fund and their co-insured family dependants. A total of 35.8 million members were covered by compulsory health insurance in 1982 (Table 7).

Table 7. CHI memberschip in 1982, broken down according to type of fund (Source: CHI statistics)

Type of health insurance fund	Comprising: No. of members (in thousands)	Non-pensioned insured (in thousands)	Pensioned insured (in thousands)
0	1	2	3
1 Local social	16 396	10 755	5 641
2 Employer	4 267	2 888	1 379
3 Artisans'	1 879	1 581	318
4 Agricultural	835	487	348
5 Seamen's	59	44	15
5 Miners'	990	337	653
7 Workmen's substitute	475	389	86
8 Salaried employees' substitute	10 916	8 954	1 962
9 Total	35 817	25 415	10 402

The relative proportion of expenditure for individual types of benefits in the total 1982 benefit expenditure of the CHI system was:

- Hospitalization, 29.6 billion DM = 31.9%
- Out-patient medical care, 16.9 billion DM = 18.3%
- Dental treatment, including dental prostheses, 13.2 billion DM = 14.3%
- Disability income benefits, 6.9 billion DM = 6.4%
- Prescribed drugs, dressings, medicines and aids, 5.4 billion DM = 5.4%
- Miscellanous benefits, 8.3 billion DM = 8.9%

The registered, full-time CHI out-patient physician (*vollzugelassener Kassenarzt*) is the basic provider of out-patient CHI medical services. He is self-employed in his own private practice (i.e. doctor's office) and therefore has full financial responsibility for the practice. Every licensed physician who satisfies the criteria for registration is legally entitled to registration as a full time CHI out-patient physician. Hospital physicians with specialist certification can also enter CHI out-patient medical practice on a part-time basis through official CHI registration, although their admission is subject to the following restrictions which do not apply to registered, full-time CHI out-patient physicians:

- Unlike CHI registration of non-hospital physicians, registration of a hospital physician with specialist certification is dependent on the existence of a need for out-patient care for CHI members.
- An application by a certified hospital doctor to participate in CHI out-patient practice must be accompanied by a statement by the physician's hospital owner/operator to the effect that such participation would not detract from the provision of in-patient care.
- Participation by a hospital doctor in CHI practice is always restricted to out-patient practice.
- A hospital physician registered for part-time CHI out-patient practice can only provide CHI out-patient care to patients referred to him by a physician admitted to CHI practice.

The associations of CHI physicians are empowered to authorize additional physicians or medically supervised facilities to provide CHI out-patient medical services in cases where the adequate provision of CHI medical services cannot be ensured by the associations' members (Table 8).

The associations of CHI physicians have also been given the responsibility of monitoring the efficiency of the provision of CHI medical care. The purposes of checking the services rendered and the prescriptions and medical certificates produced by CHI out-patient physicians are as follows:

- Verification of the arithmetic of changes calculated and of compliance with the official scales of medical fees, and adjustment where appropriate
- Counselling of the physician regarding efficient methods of treatment and prescription
- Verification of adherence to the principle of efficiency in the provision of medical care for which fees are submitted, and adjustment where appropriate
- Deciding on claims submitted by health insurance funds regarding uneconomic prescription practices

In keeping with the general obligation to secure the provision of CHI out-patient medical care, the associations of CHI physicians have utilized their by-laws to introduce certain

Table 8. Physicians engaged in CHI out-patient practice, broken down according to field of medicine and type of admission to CHI practice on 31 December 1982 (Source: national physicians' register of the National Association of Compulsory Health Insurance Physicians)

	Type of physician	Total physicians (cols. 2 to 14)	Including the following physicians admitted to CHI out patient medical practice through		
			Registration (full-time; in accord. with art. 24 of the Rules and Regulations and art. 5 , § 5, of the SHIFC)	Registration (part-time; in accord. with art. 29 of the Rules and Regulations and art. 5, 6 of the SHIFC)	Only authorization (in accord. with art. 31 of the Rules and Regulations and art. 3, § 5a, of the SHIFC)
		No.	No.	No.	No.
1	Ophthalmologists	3 023	2 949	39	35
2	Surgeons	2 782	1 395	1 103	284
3	Gynaecologists	5 905	5 138	469	298
4	Otorhinolaryngologists	2 304	2 205	60	39
5	Dematologists	1 667	1 610	17	40
6	Internists	11 285	9 371	1 098	816
7	Paediatricians	3 655	2 993	179	483
8	Laboratory specialists	464	263	56	145
9	Pneumonologists	418	347	40	31
10	Neuropyschiatrists	2 880	1 648	163	1 069
11	Orthopaedics	2 458	2 297	116	45
12	Radiologists	1 696	1 155	439	102
13	Urologists	1 477	1 269	150	58
14	Other specialists[a]	1 789	376	144	1 269
15	Total specialists, not including certified GPs[b]	41 803	33 016	4 073	4 714
16	Certified GPs	12 440	12 309	–	131
17	Non-certified GPs	14 053	13 197	11	845
18	Total GPs	26 493	25 506	11	976
19	Total physicians (15 + 18)	68 296	58 522	4 084	5 690

[a] Including anaesthetists, child psychiatrists, maxillofacial surgeons, pathologists, nuclear medicine specialists, pharmacologists, and occupational specialists.

[b] Not including general practitioners in the public health services and forensic medicine specialists.

measures designed to maintain the quality of medical services (e.g. laboratory services, cytological tests, x-ray services). These measures are binding for all physicians who provide CHI out-patient medical care. For example, quality control of laboratory services is achieved through rotating inter-laboratory trials, and quality control of x-ray services through examinations by an x-ray commission.

Drugs are the most frequent therapeutic measure prescribed by physicians. Thus, in 1981, CHI physicians wrote 421 million prescriptions for 818 million drugs for CHI patients. The total value of prescriptions amounted to 14.5 billion DM, based on retail prices. In order to aid CHI out-patient physicians in evaluating the economy of their prescription practices, the National Committee of CHI Physicians and CHI Funds (*Bundesausschuß der Ärzte und Krankenkassen*) prepared a price comparison list of drugs (*Preisvergleichsliste*) which is compiled in such a manner that the physician is able to compare prices and select prescription sizes which are appropriate to the respectice therapy.

The list is constantly updated, and the current one comprises only single-agent preparations. Uniform criteria have not been established for multi-agent preparations.

The drug guidelines of the National Committee of CHI Physicians and CHI Funds list a number of drugs which must not be prescribed at all, or only under certain conditions, for out-patient treatment at the expense of a CHI fund. Such pharmaceutical include weight-reducing preparations, cellular therapeutics, roborants, tonics, ablactation drugs (unless medically indicated), geriatric preparations (when they are intended to influence the physiological effects of aging) and vitamin preparations (except in the case of vitamin deficiency).

The hospitals in the Federal Republic of Germany provide in-patient medical care for persons covered by private or compulsory health insurance. The guiding principles in providing hospital services are need satisfaction und public interest. The small number of privately owned hospitals are an exception in that they are operated by their owners for profit (Table 9). On 31 December 1981, there were 3206 hospitals with a total of 702834 beds. Of these, 1952 were hospitals for acute cases and 1254 were special hospitals.

The number of hospitals has been declining since 1977, with the major decrease in those with fewer than 100 beds. The closing of such hospitals has particularly involved small rural institutions that provided in-patient medical care which covered a large geographical area and was patient-friendly, relative-friendly and uniform. As a result of the trend towards the closing of small hospitals, average hospitals size has increased. In addition, the remaining large hospitals are almost exclusively institutions operated by public owners. In view of the different types of owner/operators, hospitals in the Federal Republic of Germany are classified according to whether they are public, independent non-profit or private hospitals.

Since 1972, regional hospital planning has been the domain of the states. It is carried out in close co-operation with the German Hospital Association, the national associations of CHI funds, regional governmental associations and the respective state committee of the National Association of PHI Funds. The goal is to develop an integrated multi-hospital system involving a division of tasks, i.e. the provision of basic, regular and maximum hospital care.

The Hospital Finance Law (*Krankenhausfinanzierungsgesetz*) provided that the total costs of a hospital be broken down into investment (ca. 15%) and operating expenses. The current Hospital Finance Law grants hospitals a legal right to receive per diem payments which fully cover operating costs and are calculated on a uniform cost-price basis. This

Table 9. Hospital statistics, 31 December 1981 (Source: Federal Bureau of Statistics)

Hospitals	3 206
hospitals for acute cases	1 952
special hospitals	1 254
Hospital beds	702 834
in hospitals for acute cases	473 804
in special hospitals	229 030
Hospital patients treated	11.6 million
in hospitals for acute cases	10.0 million
in special hospitals	1.6 million
Days of hospitalization	213.7 million
in hospitals for acute cases	142.4 million
in special hospitals	71.3 million
Average length of hospital stay	19.4 days
in hospitals for acute cases	14.7 days
in special hospitals	51.2 days
Average rate of bed utilization	84.2%
in hospitals for acute cases	82.3%
in special hospitals	88.1%

system has not functioned adequately, and an amendment to the Hospital Finance Law is currently in preparation.

The number of physicians and male and female nurses working in hospitals has increased substantially in the past 20 years. In 1960, approximately 23 000 physicians were employed in hospitals, compared to nearly 67 500 in 1981. The number of male and female nurses rose from 110 000 to 252 000 during the same period (Table 10).

Public health services constitute the third major branch of the health care system in the Federal Republic of Germany, which supplements the work of hospital physicians and those in private practice. Public health services fulfil their responsibility of preserving the health of the population, particularly through public health protection and provision of public health benefits. This branch of the health care system is accordingly entrusted with the implementation of numerous federal and state health laws. The most important tasks of the public health services include:

- Supervision of proper training of non-academic health professionals
- Lobbying for provision of facilities necessary for public health care
- Prevention and combating of contagious human diseases
- Attention to the health aspects of environmental protection, including radiation protection
- Supervision of the drug and narcotics trade, and of the marketing of poisons and poisonous pesticides
- Provision of health benefits through counselling and supply of health services to sections of the public which require special services, and provision of school health and dental services
- Provision of official medical opinions

Table 10. Hospital personnel breakdown as of 31 December 1981

Total number of doctors		74 656
Full-time doctors	67 527	
Full-time dentists		963
Nursing personnel (not including trainees)		285 293
Nurses	187 520	
Paediatric nurses	23 519	
Nursing assistants	39 262	
Paediatric nursing assistants	1 757	
Other health care workers (without specialized training)	33 235	
Nursing personnel trainees		73 270
Midwives (including trainees)		6 481
Pharmacists		4 570
Medical technical personnel		45 829
Physiotherapists, masseurs		14 991
Other personnel		29 156
Administration and management personnel		239 976
Total		775 135
Total number of regular beds	702 834	
Per doctors	9.4	
Per nurse (not including trainees)	2.5	
Per administration and management personnel	2.9	

Source: Statistisches Bundesamt.

The organization and implementation of public health services is the responsibility of the states.

The public health offices are the central authorities for all governmental health efforts at the local administrative level. They have been set up like lower-level public authorities, as special agencies in small towns and minicipal regions. The head of a public health office is a public health officer (Table 11). The main functions of public health officers are outlined below:

1. Functions prescribed by the Law on the Interstate-Standardization of the Health Care System (*Gesetz über die Vereinheitlichung des Gesundheitswesens*), including, in particular, maintenance of practice location records; supervision of medical duties of medical officers; preparation of official medical opinions by medical legal officers; superivison of medical personnel; professional monitoring of the operation of pharmacies, and of the trade in drugs; poinsons and narcotics; and publication of health information
2. Granting of nursing permits and permits to work as a masseur, medical bath specialist, medical technician or physiotherapist; monitoring of emergency life-saving and patient-transport systems
3. Epidemic control and other functions specified by the Federal Epidemics Law (*Bundesseuchengesetz*); decontamination of buildings and objects

Table 11. Public health office personnel in 1981 (Source: Federal Bureau of Statistics)

Public health offices		320
Personnel, total		18 012
Physicians[a]	4 155	
Dentists[b]	1 878	
Health inspectors	997	
Disinfectors	242	
Medico-technical personnel[c]	690	
Social workers	2 488	
Physician's assistants[d]	1 197	
Other personnel including administrative staff[e]	6 365	

a Full-time and part-time physicians (2 282 full-time physicians in 1981).
b Full-time and part-time dentists (320 full-time dentists in 1981).
c Including medico-technical, laboratory and radiology personnel).
d Including male and female and paediatric nurses.
e Including health engineers (ca. 58)
socio-medical assistants (ca. 485)
dental assistants (ca. 330).

4. Medical duties involved in: urban hygiene; water and waste materials hygiene; noise control; water pollution control; and radiation control
5. Vaccination
6. Health benefits (*Gesundheitshilfe*): youth and school medical care; postnatal health guidance; school sports medical care; school dental care and regular dental examination and monitoring of infants and children of school age; kindergarten medical care; health services of tuberculosis patients and those exposed to tubercular infection, the mentally ill, the physically and/or mentally handicapped, those with speech defects (incuding therapeutic pedagogic services), and those with venereal diseases; constant monitoring and detection of the sources of venereal infection as prescribed by law
7. Official social service duties (*Sozialdienst*)
8. Tuberculosis income-support benefits
9. Health resort and convalescence services for children and adults
10. Preparation of medical statistics and other health reports

3.3 Guideline Medical Data

In contemplating the future development of the health care system in the Federal Republic of Germany, consideration must be given to medical science developments in the areas of prevention, diagnostics, therapy and nursing. Increasing use of electronic data processing and personal computers or terminals must be expected in all these areas. Electronic data processing can particularly be applied to the rationalization and improvement of patient care; computer-directed monitoring and therapy; integrated processing of medical data in laboratory, hospital ward and administrative areas; and the organization of long-term follow-up care.

Investigation of various models has been under way in the Federal Republic of Germany for a number of years in order to promote the further development of primary prevention. In view of the growing magnitude expenditure on treatment of disorders attributable to self-destructive behaviour, the significance of primary prevention is increasing irrespective of the fact that the health-consicious behvaiour of a given individual cannot decisively influence environmental factors or a genetically related predisposition.

In the Report on Guideline Medical Data (*Medizinische Orientierungsdaten*) submitted to the Joint Commission on the Health Care System in March 1983 by the German Medical Association (the association of state-level West German medical associations), expansion and continued development of genetic counselling and prenatal diagnostics were stated to be absolutely essential. Other measures considered to be of continuing necessity were inoculation against tetanus, diphtheria, measles and German measles, mumps and polio, as well as the introduction of other inoculations, e.g. against hepatitis B.

In addition to the existing measures for early diagnosis of disease, increased measures for early detection of cancer are needed, as well as increased efforts for early detection and treatment of hypertension.

In the area of diagnostics, future developments will favour procedures with minimal danger to the patient, and maximum objectivity, specificity and sensitivity. In the fields of clinical chemistry and pathology, new development and increased use of biochemical, immunochemical and radiochemical laboratory methods, tumour markers and histological, histochemical, immunohistochemical and electron-microscopical procedures can be expected. Equipment of rapid determination of important metabolic parameters (electrolytes, pH, acid-base balance, blood glucose, etc.) will be required, especially for intensive-care medicine and very sophisticated surgery.

The revokution in pictorial techniques brought about by the introduction of computer-assisted X-ray tomography will continue.

The development of artificial organ therapy will also continue, with extracorporal or intracorporal prosthetic applications designed to support, relieve or replace failing or functionally disturbed organs. The significance of destruction of pathological structures with the aid of sound waves should continue to increase. Despite the success of chemotherapy in the treatment of certain tumours, radiotherapy and surgical treatment will continue to be of great importance in the treatment of cancerous diseases.

Efforts for the further reduction of hospitals stays will continue. Initiatives to that end which call for maximum out-patient treatment wherever possible will continue to increase. There are, however, medical, legal and structural limits to such efforts. As in other countries, it will also be necessary to introduce a system of multiple levels of medical care in the Federal Republic of Germany on a mid- and long-term basis. There is a substantial shortage of services in individual branches of health care, obstetrics and psychiatry.

Greece

A. Kalandidi and A. Ritsataki

1 Present Position of Physicians in Greece

1.1 Total Supply of Physicians

As can be seen from Table 1, there was a rise in the rate of increase in the number of physicians during the 1970s, compared to the previous decade.

At the present time, there are about 27 600 physicians in Greece for a population of 9 850 000. Thus, with a ratio of less than 360 inhabitants per physician, the supply of doctors in Greece in relation to the total population is one of the highest in the world.

1.2 Specialisation and Regional Distribution

As can be seen from Table 2, however, the regional distribution of physicians is extremely uneven, 57% of all physicians being situated in Greater Athens and a further 15% in Salonika.

Although the ratio of inhabitants to physicians has improved in practically all regions of the country over the past 20 years, the regional distribution of physicians has not. In some areas, the improvement of the inhabitants to physician ratio has been due more to a reduction in the population in those areas than to success in attracting medical manpower.

Table 1. Number of physicians in Greece, 1960–1983

1960	10 424	1970	14 263	1980	23 469
1961	10 423	1971	14 883	1981	24 724
1962	10 723	1972	15 351	1982	25 909
1963	11 265	1973	16 984	1983	27 607
1964	11 980	1974	17 942		
1965	12 072	1975	18 421		
1966	12 383	1976	19 340		
1967	12 839	1977	20 484		
1968	13 159	1978	21 320		
1969	13 712	1979	22 337		

Source: Statistical Yearbooks, National Statistical Service.

Table 2. Inhabitants per physician, by geographical region, 1960, 1970, 1980

Gegographical region	Inhabitants per physician			Indices	
	1960	1970	1980	1970	1980
Total Greece	805	615	415		
Greater Athens	500[a]	338	226	1.0	1.0
Central Greece and Euboea	2000[a]	1290	1330	3.8	5.9
Peloponnese	1301	1010	853	3.0	3.8
Ionian Islands	1436	1175	1009	3.5	4.5
Epirus	1959	1116	845	3.3	3.8
Thessaly	1497	1176	760	3.5	3.4
Mecedonia	1106	672	424	2.0	1.9
Thrace	2764	1263	809	3.7	3.6
Aegean Islands	1197	878	875	2.6	3.9
Crete	1252	988	779	2.9	3.5

Source: Statistical Yearbooks of Greece, 1961, 1971, 1981; Population censuses 1961, 1971, 1981.
[a] Estimated figure (there was a change in the boundaries of these two regions after 1960).

In Tables 3 and 4, the regional distribution of physicians in four broad categories is presented. These categories are (a) non-specialists; (b) medical specialists (neuropsychiatrists, cardiologists, paeditricians, tuberculosis specialists, gastro-enterologists and dermatologists); (c) surgical specialists (obstetricians, gynaecologists, surgeons, thoracic surgeons, orthopaedists, urologists, ophthalmologists, otorhinolaryngologists, neurosurgeons, paediatric surgeons and anaesthesiologists); and (d) laboratory specialists (microbiologists, radiologists and medial jurisprudents).

As can be seen from Table 3, over 60% of all physicians are specialists. This seemingly high proportion, however, needs some explaining.

Owing to the way in which the health services have been organised in Greece up to the present time, most patients make a self-diagnosis of their ailment and, on this basis, visist

Table 3. Physicians by broad category of specialisation and geographical region, 1980

Geographical region		Specialisation[a] of physician Total	Non-specialised	Medical	Surgical	Laboratory
Total Greece	No.	23 469	9 046	6 428	5 209	2 786
	%	100.0	38.5	27.1	22.2	11.9
Greater Athens	No.	13 408	5 026	3 693	3 017	1 672
	%	100.0	37.5	27.5	22.5	12.5
Central Greece and Euboea	No.	827	379	218	150	80
	%	100.0	45.8	26.4	18.1	9.7
Peloponnese	No.	1 187	532	285	238	132
	%	100.0	44.8	24.0	20.1	11.1
Ionian Islands	No.	181	56	61	40	24
	%	100.0	30.9	33.7	22.1	13.3
Epirus	No.	384	149	117	75	43
	%	100.0	38.8	30.5	19.5	11.2
Thessaly	No.	915	395	262	170	88
	%	100.0	43.2	28.6	18.6	9.6
Macedonia	No.	5 005	1 818	1 396	1 201	590
	%	100.0	36.3	27.9	24.0	11.8
Thrace	No.	427	212	92	84	39
	%	100.0	49.6	21.5	19.7	9.1
Aegean Islands	No.	490	217	123	98	52
	%	100.0	44.3	25.1	20.0	10.6
Crete	No.	645	262	181	136	66
	%	100.0	40.6	28.1	21.1	10.2

Source: Statistical Yearbook of Greece, National Statistical Service, 1981.

[a] Medical specialists (internists, neuropsychiatrists, cardiologists, paediatricians, tuberculosis specialists, gastro-enterologists, dermatologists) surgical specailists (obstetricians, gynaecologists, surgeons, thoracic surgeons, orthopaedists, urologists, ophthalmologists, otorhinolaryngologists, neurosurgeons, paediatric surgeons, anaesthesiologists), laboratory specialists (microbiologists, radiologists, pathologists, medical jurisprudents).

a specialist. As a result, the bulk of the work carried out by many specialists in Greece would have been carried out by a general or family doctor in most other European countries.

The grouping of physicians into broad categories (Tables 3 and 4), whilst claryfing some regional variations, tends to conceal serious aspects of the maldistribution of doctors. Some of the 53 counties in Greece have an insufficient number of physicians with certain basic specialities, e.g. anaesthesiologists, orthopaedists and psychiatrists, a fact which partly explains the very marked movement of patients from other parts of the country to Athens and Salonika for hospital treatment.

Table 4. Inhabitants per physician, by specialisation of physician and geographical region, 1980

Geographical region	Specialisation[a] of physician			
	Non-specialised	Pathology	Surgery	Laboratory
Total Greece	1 077	1 515	1 870	3 496
Greater Athens	602	820	1 003	1 811
Central Greece and Euboea	1 330	2 901	7 331	13 745
Peloponnese	1 903	3 553	4 254	7 671
Ionian Islands	3 262	2 994	4 568	7 610
Epirus	2 178	2 774	4 327	7 547
Thessaly	1 761	2 655	4 092	7 905
Macedonia	1 167	1 520	1 767	3 597
Thrace	1 628	3 752	4 110	8 852
Aegean Islands	1 975	3 484	4 373	8 241
Crete	1 917	2 774	3 693	7 609

Source: Statistical Yearbook of Greece, 1981, National Statistical Service.

[a] See footnote to Table 3.

1.3 Employment of Physicians

Of the 27 607 physicians in the country in 1983, 13 617 were employed in hospitals and clinics (both public and private)[1]. Of these, it is estimated that about 1500 are university teaching staff, 4500 are specialists and 3500 are undergoing specialised training.

About 5200 physicians are employed by the insurance organization for urban workers (IKA) as family doctors or in its primary care centres. There are about 850 insured persons per IKA doctors for primary care. A further 1500 physicians are employed by the insurance organization for the rural population (OGA), with a ratio of about 2000 patients per doctor.

Until the implementation of the National Health System, doctors employed in hospitals worked an average of 5–6 h a day (excluding days when the hospital admits casualties); under the NHS they will work a 7.5-h day. Those employed in the IKA primary care centres work about 4–5 h, and many hold other positions in private clinics or run their own private surgeries. There is no estimate of the extent of this multiple-position holding and, therefore, of the extent of the private sector. The lack of facilities in the public sector has facilitated the growth of the private sector.

The law setting up the NHS, which was passed in 1983, provides for the employment of doctors in state hospitals and health centres on a full-time and exclusive basis. Physicians employed in state hospitals and in the primary care services of the National Health System are prohibited from engaging in private practice.

Physicians currently employed by IKA and OGA and those employed in state hospitals are remunerated on a salaried basis. Physicians who are contracted to other insurance

[1] Since this chapter was written, 7000 doctors have accepted positions in NHS hospitals.

Table 5. Physicians employed in hospitals, by geographical region, 1970 and 1980

Geographical region	No. of physicians		Beds/physcian		Nurses/physician	
	1970	1980	1970	1980	1970	1980
Total Greece	6 005	11 871	9.0	5.1	2.1	1.6
Greater Athens	3 641	7 145	7.5	4.1	2.0	1.5
Central Greece and Euboae	226	309	10.6	8.3	2.0	1.8
Peloponnese	322	589	10.9	6.4	2.2	1.8
Ionian Islands	64	109	17.1	10.0	2.9	2.2
Epirus	97	136	9.8	6.3	2.0	1.9
Thessaly	209	396	11.1	7.1	2.3	1.9
Macedonia	1 000	2 438	9.8	5.2	1.8	1.5
Thrace	75	196	9.9	5.8	2.0	1.7
Aegean Islands	146	217	27.5	15.1	4.5	3.2
Crete	225	345	11.1	8.3	2.3	2.1

Source: Social Welfare and Health Statistics, 1970 and 1980, National Statistical Service.

organisations are remunerated on a free-for-service or free-for-consultation basis, either directly by the insurance organisation or by the patient.

1.4 Monitoring of Medical Practice

There has so far been very little provision in Greece for monitoring of the quality of medical services. Unlike medical associations in some other countries, the Greek medical associations have not untertaken peer group evaluation, neither do they issue to their members any guides for medical standards.

In many countries, medical audit or tissue committees monitor the quality of medical care in hospitals. As yet such committees have not been set up in Greek hospitals. Article 12 of the law setting up the NHS provices for "scientific committees" in hospitals. The responsibilities of these committees, however, seem to be related more to organizational questions and to the in-service training of physicians than to the monitoring of services. According to a law passed in December 1985, the scientific committees can also propose the establishment of "hospital infections committees", and a central committee to study incidents of cross-infections in hospitals and to issue the necessary policy guidelines has been set up in the Ministry of Health, Welfare and Social Insurance. Although, therefore, monitoring activities have not yet become general practice in Greece, there are some indications of their gradual introduction. In addition, to the above provisions which have been made in hospitals, IKA, for example, has in recent years introduced a system for the monitoring of drug prescription.

1.5 Social Background of Physicians

Some indication of the social background of physicians in Greece can be obtained by examining the background of medical students over the past 20 years. From Table 6, which gives the number of medical students according to their parents' place of permanent residence, it can be seen that during the 2 previous decades about 60% of medical students whose parents were living in Greece were from Greater Athens of Macedonia. This must partly explain the reluctance of graduates to serve in rural areas.

As Table 7 indicates, the majority of medical students come from agricultural and working-class families, only about 20% having fathers who are in professional, managerial or high-level administrative positions.

The educational level of the fathers of medical students reveals a similar picture. In 1978–1979, for example, 28% of medical students had fathers who were themselves university graduates; a further 28% of fathers had completed secondary school, 34% had completed primary school, 8% had not completed primary school and 1% were illiterate.

1.6 Age and Sex Structure of Medical Manpower

Data on the age and sex structure of the members of the medical profession can be obtained from the Annual Survey of Employment, which is carried out by the National Statistical Service. These data reveal that approximately 35% of physicians are women,

Table 6. Medical students, by their parents' place of permanent residence

Parents' residence	Medical students					
	1960–1961		1969–1970		1978–1979	
	No.	%	No.	%	No.	%
Greater Athens[a]	879	29.3	2 636	37.6	2 409	43.0
Central Greece and Euboea	190	6.3	456	6.5	423	7.6
Peloponnese	321	10.7	588	8.4	497	8.9
Ionian Islands	41	1.4	144	2.1	99	1.8
Epirus	83	2.8	178	2.5	150	2.7
Thessaly	206	6.9	430	6.1	378	6.8
Macedonia	935	31.1	1 870	26.7	1 036	18.4
Thrace	62	2.1	149	2.1	84	1.5
Aegean Islands	116	3.9	177	2.5	158	2.8
Crete	163	5.4	315	4.5	244	4.4
No reply	2	0.1	66	0.9	116	2.1
Total Greece	2 998	100.0	7 009	100.0	5 594	100.0
Abroad[b]	217	(6.7)	1 259	(15.2)	1 333	(19.2)

Source: Aducation Statistics, 1960–1961, 1969–1970, 1978–1979, National Statistical Service.

[a] 1960–1961 refers to the county of Attica.
[b] % total students.

Table 7. Medical students, by father's occupation in acadmic years 1960–1961, 1969–1970, 1978–1979

Father's occupation	Medical students 1960–1961		1969–1970		1978–1979	
	No.	%	No.	%	No.	%
Professional	669	20.9	1338	16.1	1476	21.2
Managerial	17	0.5	172	2.1	75	1.1
Clerical	327	10.2	1205	14.6	1232	17.8
Trade and commerce	402	12.5	1222	14.8	1071	15.5
Agriculture and fishing	570	17.7	1537	18.5	866	12.5
Manufacturing, transport and communications	370	11.5	1303	15.8	1155	16.7
Services, recreation	80	2.5	235	2.8	368	5.3
Other non-specified	29	0.9	14	0.2	14	0.2
Armed forces	39	1.2	188	2.3	290	4.2
Pensioners, not gainfully employed	328	10.2	785	9.5	191	2.8
No reply	384	11.9	269	3.3	189	2.7
Total	3215	100.0	8268	100.0	6927	100.0

Source: *Education Statistics*, 1960–1961, 1969–1970, 1978–1979, National Statistical Service.

and this proportion does not vary to any great extent between urban and rural areas. About 33% of all physicians are under the age of 35, and more than 8% are 60 or over. In rural areas, the proportion of physicians aged 60 or over is slightly higher.

1.7 Migration of Physicians

In recent years, the National Statistical Service has discontinued the collection of detailed data on those entering and leaving the country. There are no reliable data, therefore, on the number of physicians immigrating or emigrating.

2 Manpower Planning and Medical Education

2.1 Manpower Planning

As can be seen from the above analysis, the maldistribution of physicians, both geographically and with regard to their specialization, is not a new phenomenon. Almost 20 years ago, in the 1966–1970 Draft Plan for the Economic Development of Greece[2], it was

2 *Draft Plan for the Economic Development of Greece 1966–1970* (1965) Centre of Planning and Economic Research, Athens, p 417 (in Greek).

pointed out that although the total number of physicians was sufficient, there was need for a considerable redistribution of doctors in favour of the provinces and an improvement in the structure from the point of view of specialisation. It was proposed at that time, that in the short-term 1000 physicians should be moved from the Greater Athens area to the provinces, by means of a system of financial incentives and the enhancement of working conditions in provincial hospitals. In the long-term, young physicians were to be attracted to the provinces by means of a scholarship system which was to be tied to provincial service.

A number of development plans have been prepared since that time, all of which indicate the same problem. Indeed, by the time that the 1976–1980 plan was formulated, the problem was considered to have become so acute that it was stated, "the total supply of physicians has already reached a level where it is detrimental to the quality of health services, due to excessive competition."[3]

Unfortunately, however, very little action was actually taken. Similar wishes were expressed throughout the 20-year period regarding the need for an improvement in the physical and technical facilities of provincial hospitals and rural clinics in order to attract physicians to those areas, but the slight improvements which have taken place have been woefully inadequate. Some differentiation was made in the renumeration of physicians in rural areas, for example, between physicians serving in mountainous and non-mounainous areas.

A law passed 20 years ago, which is still in effect, provided for compulsory services by medical school graduates in rural clinics. This has had the effect of keeping open the rural surgeries, but has meant that the rural population is provided with a low level of health care by inexperienced young physicians, cut off from their more experienced colleagues. It was recently announced that this regulation is to remain in effect for the next 5 years at least.

During the 1967–1974 dictatorship, an attempt was made to restrict the medical school intake and to prevent the transfer of medical students from foreign universities to Greek medical schools. Notwithstanding the restrictions on freedom of speech in force at the time, public protest at these proposals was so great that they were abandoned.

Various other measurements, which were considered would attract physicians to the provinces, were suggested throughout this period, such as declaring the Medical Associations in certain large towns to have reached full capacity; linking the services of rural clinics and state hospitals; employing hospital doctors on a full-time basis; and setting up medical schools in provincial universities. Only the last of these measures was implemented, medical schools being established in Patras, Jannina, Crete and Thrace.

The problems posed in the field of health planning with regard to medical manpower were not, however, related to educational planning. The failure to related health manpower planning to planning for the education of physicians is not restricted simply to the number and specialization of doctors being produced. It is something more basic.

Firstly, there has been a failure adequately to define the role of the physician in the health services, insufficient attention having been given to the role of the physician in the health team. This obviously has an impact on the content of medical education; indeed,

---

3 *Health*. Report of Workung Group for Health, 1976–1980 Development Plan (1976) Centre of Planning and Economic Research, Athens, p 265 (in Greek).

until recently the educational programme made no provision, for example, for the future "social" role of the physician or for the physicians's relationship with the other members of the health team. This has not only detrimental consequences for the overall effectiveness and efficiency of the health team but also an immediate impact on the number of medical personnel needed for the health services.

To clarify this point, it may be mentioned that physicians in Greece can be observed carrying out activities which in other countries would be the function of the nursing or administrative personnel of the health services. Obviously, this has a considerable effect on the total number of physicians "needed" or, conversely, can be seen as a consequence of the unplanned growth in the supply of physicians.

The internist in Greece is used by the population as a general or family doctor, although his training does not really fit him for this task. Although there has been repeated reference throughout the last 20 years to the need for a "family doctor", it is only with the educational programme which has been set up for community medicine in the medical school in Greece and the recent establishment of specialization in general medicine that any attempt has been made to adapt the medical education system to meet that need.

Although Greece has one of the most rapidly aging populations in Europe (persons aged 60 or over accounted for 17.7% of the population in 1980; and this proportion is expected to have risen to 21.1% by the year 2000), medical education has not been adapted to give more attention to the care of the elderly and to the increasing importance of chronic diseases.

On the whole, Greek medical schools lack sufficient technical equipment and facilities, laboratories, etc. It has been said[4] that this fact has been instrumental in shaping medical education, i.e. there has been a tendency to adjust the aims of medical education to fit the means available, with consequently greater emphasis on theoretical education, rather than to adjust medical education to meet specific aims related to the needs of the health services.

There has been no attempt at carrer guidance with regard to the postgraduate education or specialisation of Greek physicians. Medical graduates have tended to choose their field of specialization mainly the the basis of popularly held beliefs as to the likely remuneration in certain specialities, and the positions available in hospitals for specialization. Similarly, the number of positions for specialization have not been geared to the needs of the health services for different types of specialities.

Finally, there has been no attempt to encourage the systematic continuing education of physicians by linking a part of their remuneration or their carreer prospects to such education, as is done in the United Kingdom, for example.

2.2 Medical Education

There are six medical schools in Greece: Athens, Salonika, Patras, Jannina, Alexandoupolis and Crete. In the academic year 1980–1981, there were 7046 students in medical schools

---

4 *Regionalisation of the Health Services.* Report of the Working Group on Health, Regional Plan for Greece, Centre of Planning and Economic Research, Athens, 1979, p 156 (in Greek).

in Greece, about 30% of whom were women. The schools in Athens and Salonika account for about 80% of all medical students.

The distribution of students was as follows:

1st year	744	4th year	963
2nd year	929	5th year	1063
3rd year	1090	6th year	950
		graduates	1307

Students are admitted to medical schools on the basis of entrace examinations, and the number to be admitted each year is set by the Ministry of Education. The considerable fluctuations in the number of students (see above) are the result of the admittance of certain categories of students without examination, e.g. students whose parents live abroad, and the transfer of students from foreign universities. Entrance into foreign universities, particularly in countries such as Italy where this is achieved without entrance examinations, followed later by transfer to Greek univerisities, has consistently been used as a means of entering Greek medical schools through the back-door. Obviously, this has serious effects on the quality of the education which can be offered. However, admission with the above-mentioned exceptions, to medical school is based solely on academic achievements.

3 Future Trends

It is rather difficult to predict future trends in the Greece medical profession in view of the radical changes taking place both in the delivery of health services and in the provision of higher level education. Although the general outline of these changes is already apparent, it is not yet clear exactly how some of them are to be implemented.

As mentioned above, a National Health System is being set up, in the framework of which state hospital services will be organised on a regional basis and linked to primary care through a network of health centres in both urban and ural areas. In addition to primary care, the health centres are expected to provide a variety of other services, e.g. family planning and support facilities for special groups such as the handicapped and the elderly. There are also expected to be basic units for the provision of preventive health. Linkes to the health centres will be a network of family doctors. Access to specialised services within the National Health System will be through referal from a general practitioner or family doctors, or through the outpatient clinics of state hospitals.

Although the health services are to be organised on a regional basis, responsibility for their provision will remain with the central government, and they will be financed entirely by central funds. Provision has been made, however, for the participation of the local authorities in the administration of the services at all levels.

Physicians employed in the National Health System are to be remunerated on a salary basis. They are to be employed full-time and will not have the right to private practice.

A National Health Council, the majority of whose members are from the medical profession, was recently set up for the planning of health policy. It will eventually be supported by a multidisciplinary secretariat. A network of regional councils, on which the local authorities will be presented, is also to be set up.

Note: This chapter was originally written in 1983. In revising it in 1986, an attempt was made to take into account legal changes and new statistics available at that time. It should be noted, however, that with the rapid changes taking place during the implementation of the NHS, some of the information is becoming out-of-date even as it is written.

Appendix. Statistical Publications

1. *Statistical Yearbook of Greece.* Published by the National Statistical Service of Greece.
   Data are compiled by the Athens and Panhellenic Medical Associations, and the Social Policy Centres of the Ministry of Health and Welfare. The number of doctors and dentists is given, by regional distribution and speciality.

2. *Bulletin of Health and Welfare Statistics.* Published annually by the National Statistical Service of Greece.
   This gives the number of physicians employed in state hospitals, health centres (only centres with beds for private health care) and private clinics. Data are given by specialisation of hospital, size of hospital and specialisation of physicians.

3. *Education Statistics.* Published annually by the National Statistical Service of Greece.
   This gives data on the number and sex of students in medical schools, their place of birth, place of residence and occupation, and the educational level of their parents.

4. *Annual Employment Survey.* Published by the National Statistical Service of Greece.
   By special request, data can be obtained from this survey on the number and sex of physicians, by age group, urban, semi-urban and rural areas, and geographical region.

Ireland

A. Walsh

The Department of Health formulates health policy and supervises the eight health boards and other executive agencies in the provision of health services. The population of Ireland is 3 443 405 (1981 census).

1 Eligibility for Health Services

Some people have entitlement to all health services, while the entitlement of others is limited to selected services. A person's eligibility for services is determined by the category to which he belongs. There are three categories.

Category 1. This category comprises persons with full eligibility, i.e. persons who, in the opinion of the Chief Executive Officer of the relevant health board, are unable to afford general practitioner services for themselves and their dependents. Persons in this group are entitled to the full range of health services without charge, and medical cards are issued to them for presentation when services are needed. Somewhat less than 40% of the population are in this category.

Category 2. This category comprises persons other than those in Category 1 whose income in the year ended 5 April 1983 was less than Ir £ 11 000 (this limit will be reviewed in future years). Persons in this category are entitled without charge to hospital services (both maintenance and treatment) in public wards, to specialist services in out-patient clinics (other than dental, ophthalmic and aural out-patient services) and to maternity and infant welfare services. They are also entitled to a refund of part of the cost of prescribed medicines. About 45% of the population are in this category.

Category 3. This category comprises persons whose income in the year ended 5 April 1983 was Ir £ 11 000 or more. Persons in this category are entitled without charge to hospital services on the same basis as those in Category 2, except that they will be liable to pay hospital consultants' fees. They are also entitled to a refund of part of the cost of prescribed medicines. Somewhat more than 15% of the population are in this category.

Where a husband and wife have separate incomes, the eligibility of each will be assessed separately. If the income of each is within the limit of Ir £ 11 000, both they and their children will be eligible for Category 2 services. The dependants of a person (i.e. husband or wife) who have no indenpendent income or who have children under 16 years of age will be in the same category for eligibility purposes as that person. If either parent is in Category 3, the dependent children will normally also be regarded as being in that category.

Hospital services for infectious diseases are available without charge to persons in all categories, and hospital in-patient and out-patient services are also available without charge for all children under 16 years of age suffering from certain long-term ailments.

A general medical service is available to those in Category 1. This entitles a person, free of charge, to the services of his chosen doctor and to obtain drugs, medicines and appliances prescribed by that doctor, usually from a local pharmacist.

A Voluntary Health Insurance Board was established under the Voluntary Health Insurance Act, 1957 to provide non-profit making health insurance schemes.

2 Undergraduate Medical Education

There are five medical schools in Ireland:

1. University College Cork. The National University of Ireland (UCC)
2. University College Dublin. The National University of Ireland (UCD)
3. University College Galway. The National University of Ireland (UCC)
4. Trinity College, University of Dublin (TCD)
5. Royal College of Surgeons in Ireland (RCSI)

Undergraduate medical education is the responsiblity of the Minister for Education, who is advised by the Higher Education Authority, a statutory body with responsibility for the development of higher education. The curriculum is a matter for each medical school. However, the Medical Council, the statutory body responsible for the registration of medical practitioners, has the duty from time to time to satisfy itself (a) as to the suitability of the medical education and training provided by any body in the State recognised by the Council for such purpose, and (b) as to the standards of theoretical and practical knowledge required for primary qualifications.

Following the 6-year course at the medical school and having passed a qualifying examination, the candidate is granted a primary qualification. He must then be employed for a period, at present 1 year, in a residential medical capacity in one or more hospitals approved by the Medical Council and be granted a certificate of experience by the body which awarded him his primary qualification in order to obtain a formal qualification in medicine.

The Medical Council also has the duty to ensure that the requirements relating to education and training for a formal qualification satisfy the minimum standards specified in any Directive adopted by the Council of the European Community relating to that qualification.

3 Entry to Medical School

For admission to a medical school, it is necessary to have passed the university matriculation or an equivalent examination with certain minimum grades. English, a science subject and, in some cases, mathematics are obligatory. Until the early 1960s, there was little difficulty in securing entrance to a school if one possessed the minimum qualifications and the necessary finance. However, because of increasing numbers seeking post-primary education and of rising prosperity and increased grants for tertiary education, the numbers seeking entry to medical schools began to rise. The Report of the Commission on Higher Education in 1967 stated that it could not be accepted that a place had to be found for everyone who sought to obtain a medical education and who satisfied the manimum admission requirements. With the development of the new teaching hospitals, it became necessary for the Higher Education Authority to determine the facilities for medical teaching to be incorporated in the plans, and in 1977 it established a special sub-committee to examine the issue of the number of places in the schools. The report of the sub-committee was published by the Authority in October 1978. The number of medical graduates in the years leading up to this report were:

1973 – 449
1974 – 445
1975 – 447
1976 – 470
1977 – 468
1978 – 451

The report proposed that an upper limit of 300 be placed in Irish admissions to medical schools, the quota to be introduced in the academic year 1980–1981. It also recommended a quota of non-Irish students except in the case of the Royal College of Surgeons or Ireland, whose authorities could determine the number of students to be admitted. Those quotas are as follows:

	Irish	Non-Irish
UCD	105	10
UCC	55	5
UCG	55	5
TCD	60	8
RCSI	25	8

The Minister for Education did not fully accept the number for UCC, and the number of Irish students was increased to 60.

The Higher Education Authority is again examining the question of numbers, and it is hoped that a final report will be available during 1984. In the meantime, it recommends that the entry of Irish students for 1983 remain as above, i.e. 300.

As Table 1 shows, the target of an entry of 305 Irish medical students for the academic year 1980–1981 was not met.

The number of medical graduates has not yet begun to fall, as Table 2 shows.

4 Numerus Clausus

There is a very strict limitation on entry and a very high academic standard is required. The number of applicants greatly exceeds the number of places, and only those who have done exceptionally well in the school-leaving examinations have any hope of gaining a place.

5 Postgraduate Medical Education

It has long been recognised that owing to the great increase in medical knowledge, it is not possible to teach the full range of modern medical practice to an undergraduate. The first step to remedy this situation was taken in 1954 when a compulsory internship year was added to the medical course.

Table 1. Intake of medical school students (Irish and non-Irish) 1978–1982

Year	1978–1979		1979–1980		1980–1981		1981–1982	
College	Irish	Non-Irish	Irish	Non-Irish	Irish	Non-Irish	Irish	Non-Irish
UCD	137	7	132	8	130	1	122	9
UCC	79	2	71	4	70	3	77	1
UCG	69		70	5	66	6	58	3
TCD	84	5	69	9	63	6	65	10
RCSI	45	80	40	81	53	82	48	92
Totals	414	94	382	107	382	98	370	115

Table 2. Intake of medical school students (Irish and non-Irish, male and female), 1980–1982

Year	Total	Irish Male	Female	Non-Irish
1980	446	226	146	94
1981	465	235	149	81
1982	458	240	130	88

Until the late 1960s, most postgraduate training was largely unstructered, the trainee selecting appointments which he thought would be of benefit to him before taking postgraduate certificate examinations conducted by the Universities and Royal Colleges. Irish medical education has traditionally been closely linked with that in the United Kingdom, and in the early 1970s the Irish Royal Colleges of Physicians and Surgeons joined with their sister colleges in the United Kingdom and formed Joint Higher Training Committees. These Committees inspect hospital posts to ensure that they are suitable for training, enrol trainees, supervise their training and issue a certificate of accreditation upon satisfactory completion of training. The training is, in broad terms, divided into a 3-year period of general professional training supervised by the Colleges and Universities, followed by a 4-year period of more specialised higher training supervised by the Joint Committees. At the end of this period, the doctor is certified as being competent to accept full responsibility in his chosen branch of medicine.

Following discussions initiated by the Minister for Health in 1973, it was decided to set up a central body to promote and co-ordinate postgraduate education and training. A Council for Postgraduate Medical and Dental Education and Training was established and was later to become a statutory body, the Postgraduate Medical and Dental Board, established under the Medical Practitioners Act, 1978. This Act also gave the Medical Council, which replaced the Medical Registration Council, the duty of satisfying itself as to the adequacy and suitability of postgraduate education and training provided by bodies recognised by the Council for the purposes of medical specialist training. Furthermore, it gave the Council power to establish, with the consent of the Minister for Health, a specialist register. To date, the Council has not sought to use this power.

The functions of the Postgraduate Medical and Dental Board are:

1. To promote the development of postgraduate medical and dental education and training, and to co-ordinate such development
2. To advise the Minister, after consultation with certain specified bodies and such other bodies as it may consider appropriate, on all matters, including financial matters, relating to the development and co-ordination of postgraduate medical and dental education and training (the specified bodies are: University College Cork; University College Dublin; University College Galway; The University of Dublin; The Royal College of Surgeons in Ireland; The Roxal College of Physicians of Ireland; such body or bodies as, in the opinion of the Minister for Health, represent psychiatry; such body or bodies as, in the opinion of the Minister for Health, represent general medical practice)
3. To provide career guidance for reistered medical practitioners and registered dentists.

Postgraduate education has been for many years the responsibility of the professional bodies, and the Medical Council and the Postgraduate Board accept, in principle, that programmed training should be under the immediate guidance of those bodies. They lay down the criteria and standards for training in different specialities and are responsible for the general organization and monitoring of training. The Board has recognized the following eight main Irish professional bodies as filling major roles in programmed training for doctors:

1. The Faculty of Anaesthetists of the Royal College of Surgeons in Ireland
2. The Irish Institute of General Practice

3. The Irish Committee on Higher Medical Training
4. The Institute of Obstetricians and Gynaecologists of the Royal College of Physicians of Ireland
5. The Faculty of Pathology of the Royal College of Physicians of Ireland
6. The Irish Psychiatric Training Committee
7. The Faculty of Radiologists of the Royal College of Surgeons in Ireland
8. The Irish Surgical Postgraduate Training Committee

General practice training is supervised by the Irish Institute of General Practice, which was established in 1975. In June 1983, 81 doctors had completed the 3-year training programme.

When the Commission on Higher Education reported in 1967 that it could not be accepted that a place had to be found for everyone who sought to obtain a medical qualification and who satisfied the minimum admission requirements, the concern was with the cost of medical education and not the fear of unemployment among doctors. The Irish medical schools had been producing doctors in excess of national requirements for decades. Many doctors emigrated, traditionally to the United Kingdom, the United States of America, Canada and Australia, where there was a ready market for their services. Many women doctors ceased practice on marriage or at the time of the birth of their first child. During the 1970s, owing to the greatly increased expansion of their own medical schools, the traditional outlets abroad for surplus Irish doctors began to disappear, and it is now very difficult for an Irish national to gain entry to the USA or Canada.

The 1970s witnessed a great expansion of the health services in Ireland, with an annual increase over a 10-year period of 4.8% in consultant (specialist) posts and, over an 8-year period, an annual increase of 7.5% in nòn-consultant hospital doctor posts. On account of economic circumstances, there has been a minimal increase during the 1980s and the prospects of an increase in the foreseeable future would appear to be slight. The increasing number of women graduates are no longer prepared to relinquish their careers when they start a family and are demanding part-time posts and part-time specialist training.

It is not possible to be accurate about the number of career posts in medicine to be filled in Ireland each year, but it is almost certainly under 150. Even though it is open to any doctor to establish himself in independent practice, it has been obvious to many interested individuals and bodies that Ireland is over-producing doctors in considerable numbers. The Department of Health conveyed its fears and the fears of other bodies to the Higher Education Authority, which is considering the matter. The Departments of Health and Education will, no doubt, meet after the Higher Education Authority has advised the Minister for Education, so that a policy decision can be made by the two Ministers concerned.

6 Hospital Staffing

Hospital staffing in Ireland is based on a system of consultants (specialists) an non-consultant hospital doctors. The consultant only has full clinical responsiblity for patients. Non-consultant posts are all temporary trainee ones, with their holders graded as intern (before formal qualification) house officer, registrar or senior registrar. Senior registrar posts are in recognised higher training programmes.

Comhairle na n-Ospideal (the Hospital Council), usually referred to as *Comhairle*, was established under the Health Act, 1970. Its main statutory function is to regulate the number and type of appointments of consultant medical staff and senior registrars in hospitals engaged in the provision of services under that Act. It also specifies qualifications for these appointments. Members of the *Comhairle* are appointed by the Minister for Health.

It publishes detailed statistics on the number of consultants and senior registrars in posts, and the number of vacant posts. Table 3 shows the number of consultants, by speciality, as at 1 May 1981.

The *Comhairle* also attempted to produce 3-year manpower projections up to 1981 and 1984. Table 4 shows the projected 1981 establishment and the actual 1981 establishment, from which it will be seen that the projection was reasonably accurate.

However, the projections to 1984 will not be realised, as new posts are not being created in the health services.

7 General Medical Practice

There is no compulsory specific training for general practice. Doctors entering the General Medical Service, the state-financed scheme for general practitioners services which covers about 40% of the population, are required to have 2 years' experience following basic training, 8-months in recognised hospital posts and 6 months in general practice. The Institute of General Practice has established a 3-year full-time vocational training course, comprising 2 years' hospital training and 1 year's general practice training. The present annual intake is 28 trainees.

Owing to the mixture of public and private medicine, there has never been a fully accurate picture of the number of doctors practising medicine in Ireland. Prior to the

Table 3. Number of consultants, by speciality, as at 1 May 1981

Speciality	1 No. of consultants in practice	2 No. of vacant posts	1 + 2 Establishment
Anaesthetists	132	35	167
Obstetricians/ Gynaecologists	93	10	103
Paediatricians	40	10	50
Pathologists	81	13	94
Physicians	172	26	198
Psychiatrists	157	25	182
Radiologists	73	15	88
Ophthalmic surgeons	34	4	38
Orthopaedic surgeons	37	3	40
Otolargyngologists	28	2	30
Surgeons	146	13	159
Total	993	156	1149

Table 4. Medical manpower for 1981 (projected establishment and actual establishment)

Speciality	Projected 1981 establishment		Actual 1981 establishment	Difference
Anaesthetists	163	(26)	167	+ 4
Obstetricians/ Gynaecologists	98	(8)	103	+ 5
Paediatricians	56	(15)	50	− 6
Pathologists	108	(26)	94	−14
Physicians	275	(39)	198	−17
Psychiatrists	172	(6)	182	+ 10
Radiologists	99	(24)	88	−11
Otolaryngologists	31	(4)	30	− 1
Opthalmic surgeons	39	(5)	38	− 1
Orthopaedic surgeons	40	(4)	40	0
Surgeons	159	(18)	159	0
Total	1180	(175)	1149	−31

establishment of the Medical Council under the Medical Practitioners Act, 1978, the regulatory body for doctors was the Medical Registration Council. This earlier Council was able to finance its activities through a once-off payment by doctors on initial registration, and no further payment was ever required. As one payment conferred life registration and as there was no mechanism whereby a doctor could voluntarily have his name removed from the register, the register did not give an accurate indication of the number of doctors practising in Ireland. The new enlarged Medical Council was given power, which it quickly exercised, to charge an annual fee for the retention of a doctor's name on the register. The new General Register of Medical Pracitioners showed that there are 8431 doctors fully registered (6376 men and 2055 women), and it was estimated that approximately 6500 of these are resident in Ireland. The Postgraduate Medical and Dental Board estimates that there are 4885 doctors in full-time medical practice, as follows:

<table>
<tr><td>Interns</td><td>360</td><td rowspan="4">1648</td></tr>
<tr><td>House officers</td><td>824</td></tr>
<tr><td>Registrars</td><td>442</td></tr>
<tr><td>General practice trainees</td><td>22</td></tr>
<tr><td>Consultants</td><td>1037</td><td></td></tr>
<tr><td>Community medicine</td><td>231</td><td></td></tr>
<tr><td>Academic medicine</td><td>90</td><td></td></tr>
<tr><td>Occupational medicine</td><td>15</td><td></td></tr>
<tr><td>Defence forces</td><td>30</td><td></td></tr>
<tr><td>General practice</td><td>1800</td><td></td></tr>
<tr><td>Others</td><td>34</td><td></td></tr>
</table>

The Department of Health, *Comhairle na n-Ospideal*, the Postgraduate Medical and Dental Board and other bodies have agreed that a major manpower study is required, and it is hoped that it will shortly be initiated.

The main problems encountered have been referred to in this article and centre on the over-production of medical graduates. It has also become apparent that there is an imbalance between the high number of trainee posts in hospitals and the limited career opportunities at consultant level, and, of course, the growing demand to facilitate for the increasing number of women doctors with family commitments the continuation of their careers in medicine.

Bibliography

Statistical Information relevant to the Health Services 1983 (1982) Planning Unit, Department of Health

The Health Services of Ireland (1979) Brendan Hensey, Institute of Public Administration

Medical Manpower in Ireland (1984) The Postgraduate Medical and Dental Board

Consultant Manpower in the Republic of Ireland 1978–1984 (1984) *Comhairle na n-Ospideal*

Consultant Manpower Projection up to 1981 (1981) *Comhairle na n-Ospideal*

Report of a Symposium on Career Guidance in Medicine (1982) Postgraduate Medical and Dental Board

Summary of the Health Services June 1983 (1983) The Department of Health

Italy

P.L. Morosini

1 The Italian National Health Service

The Italian National Health Service (INHS) was established in December 1978, replacing an insurance system composed of different agencies. Its structure is similar to that of the British NHS, with three different administrative levels: national, regional (20 regions) and local (the *Unità Sanitaria Locale* (USL), or local health district, such districts numbering about 650). The INHS differs from the British NHS, however, in that it is more decentralized. In fact, the USLs and the Regions have locally elected or appointed councils. USLs are directly responsible for providing preventive, curative and rehabilitation services according to regional and national plans, and within a fixed budget.

Physicians are employed directly by the INHS or have special individual contracts; or they are employed by agencies that have reimbursement contracts with the INHS. Only a small number of physicians, mainly dentists, are engaged full-time in private practice.

In the first category (physicians employed directly by the INHS) are physicians working in public hospitals and public health services. A little less than 60% of the physicians in public hospitals are employed full-time (38 hours a week), whereas the rest are employed part-time (28 hours a week) and may undertake private practice and/or serve as general practitioners or as specialists in out-patient departments (see below).

The second category (physicians contracted to the INHS) comprises general practitioners, paid on a per capita basis, and specialists in out-patient departments or services. The majority of the latter work in public out-patient facilities and are paid on an hourly basis, while a small number work on external contracts within their own practice and are paid on a fee-for-service basis when they visit INHS patients. Group practice in primary care is very rare; general practitioners with a large number of patients may, however, take on a young colleague in a subordinate position.

The third category comprises almost exclusively physicians working in private hospitals which have contracts with the INHS. They are distributed disparately and are more frequently found in the South and in the area around Rome. Of the total beds available, 84% are in hospitals directly managed by the INHS and 16% are private hospital beds contracted to the INHS; only a very small fraction of hospital beds are totally private.

2 Data Sources and Previous Studies

The main sources of information on Italian physicians are a data base manged by the National Medical Association and the routine statistics published yearly by the Central Institute of Statistics.

ENPAM, the special insurance institute for physicians, managed by the National Medical Association, registers on the Medical Association List (*Albo dell'Ordine dei Medici*) all physicians qualified to practise medicine. Although it is possible to obtain special analyses on request, no routine data are published. Unfortunately, the data base does no distinguish between practising and non-practising physicians among the different specialities or posts occupied. It should also be pointed out that almost all Italian dentists are medically qualified and are not differentiated from other physicians in this data base.

The Central Institute of Statistics provides data in the *Annuario Statistico Italiano* on the number of private and public hospitals physicians, by Region of practice and level within the hospital career pattern. The most recent data refer to 1982 (1). Data on enrolled medical students, qualifying physicians and those taking postgraduate specializations are also included in the *Annuario Statistico dell'Istruzione*, the most recent of such data unfortunately relating only to 1980 (2).

Pharmaceutical firms have carried out a number of surveys of physicians registered on client lists, but these are of course not representative.

Among the studies on medical resources in Italy, the most comprehensive were conducted by the Institute for Research into Medical Economics (*Istituto per la Ricerca di Economia Sanitaria*) (3) and Magi, Splendori and Vanini (4). Magi has also authored some ad hoc studies on the distribution of and prospects for young physicians (5).

3 Number and Geographical Distribution of Medical Resources

At the end of June 1984, 219 519 physicians were registered on the Medical Association List, i.e. 1 physician per 258 inhabitants or 3.8 physicians per 1000 population. Of these, about 8% are already entitled to draw a pension and 7% are believed to be dentists (3). There remain about 186 500 physicians, including a few employed in biological research departments or in administration. From these data, it is estimated that there are 3.3 active physicians per 1000 population or 1 active physician per 303 inhabitants.

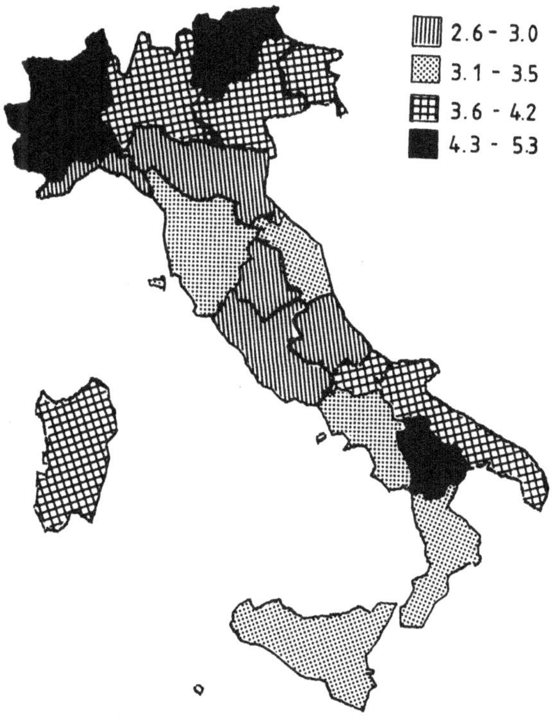

Fig. 1. Distribution of physicians per 1000 population by Region; all physicians registered in the Italian Medical Association List are included

The geographical distribution of physicians registered on the Medical Association List is not homogenous, varying from 2.6 to 5.3 physicians per 1000 population (Fig. 1), with the highest density in Lazio, in the Region of Rome. As in all other countries, there are more physicians practising in urban areas (1 physician per 148 inhabitants in provincial capital towns) than in rural areas (1 per 403 inhabitants in the remainder of the country).

4 Number and Age and Sex Distribution

During the period 1954–1984, the number of Italian physicians (Fig. 2a) almost quadrupled (rising from 60 000 to 220 000), with an increase from 1.2 to 3.8 per 1000 population (Fig. 2b). The slope of the curve began to change in 1976, when students enrolled after the 1969 "free University access" law began to complete their studies. A sharp increase in the number of students enrolled in medical schools began to occur in 1970 (Fig. 3), when, in the absence of programmed admission intake or a *numerus clausus,* access to medical schools was made open to any student with a secondary school diploma. Previously, schools had been open only to students with a diploma from a high school specializing in the sciences or the humanities.

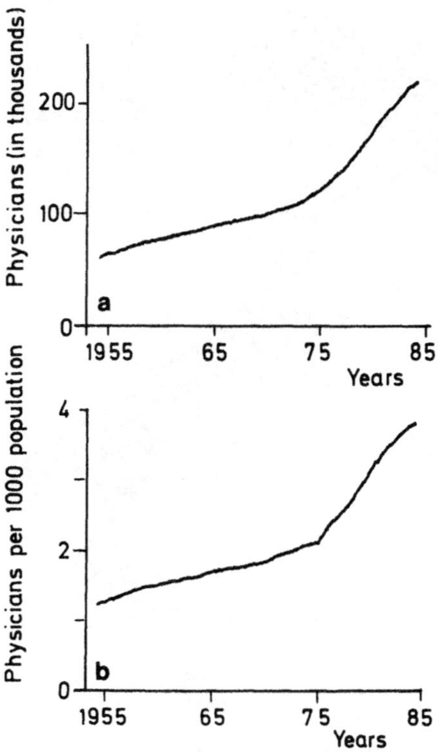

Fig. 2. a Number of physicians. **b** Physicians/population ratio in the period 1965–1984

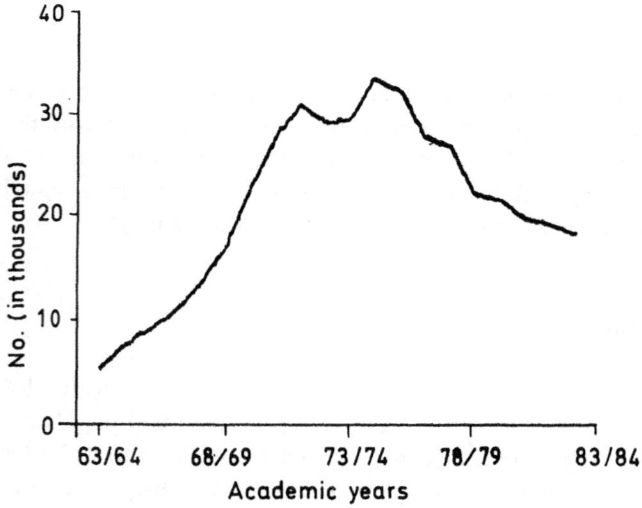

Fig. 3. Intake of first-year medical students in the period 1963–1983

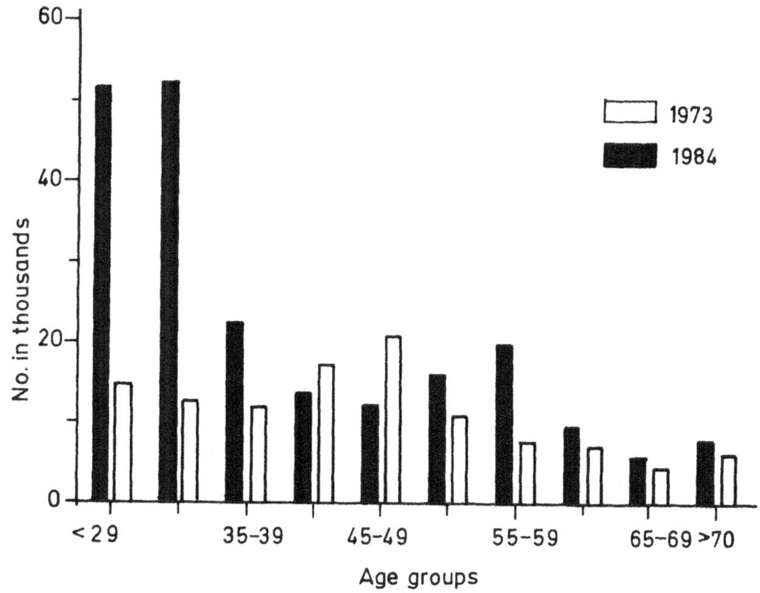

Fig. 4. Distribution of physicians by age in 1973 and 1983

The age distribution of Italian physicians is consequently skewed towards the youngest ages: whereas in 1973 less than a quarter of registered physicians were 34 years old or younger, in 1984 almost half fell into this age group (Fig. 4).

Of the physicians registered on the Medical Association List, 81% are males and 19% females. However, the proportion of women among medical graduates has increased to about 30% in recent years: in 1984, 33.5% of physicians in the 25–29 age group were women (5).

5 Medical Schools

There are 29 medical schools in Italy, of which all except one are public, and in 1982–1983 they enrolled about 160 000 students. The medical schools with the highest number of students are located in Naples, Rome and Milan, each of which has an intake of more than 2000 first-year students. In general, medical students are unevenly distributed, since six schools enrol more than 50% of the total medical student body.

Of the 160 000 students in the academic years 1982–1983, only 110 000 (69%) had passed all the basic yearly examinations, the remainder not following a full programme of study each year. This supports the estimate that only slightly more than 50% of students in medical school during the 1970s obtained medical qualifications.

Large numbers of foreign medical students, mainly from the United States, Israel and Greece, have completed studies or are studying in Italy. In 1977, there were about 10 000 foreign medical students, representing 6% of the total medical student population.

Figure 3 shows that the number of newly enrolled medical students reached about 31 000 in 1975 but dropped to 18 200 in the academic year 1983–1984. This includes about 800 students enrolled in the new programme leading to qualification in dentistry. A 40% decrease took place during the 10-year period. However, notwithstanding the large number of qualified physicians, the number of new medical students is now the same as in 1968; furthermore, the decrease rate seems to have slowed down during the last 2 years. In 1981 and in 1982, there were just over 15 000 new medical qualifications, i.e. 265 per million inhabitants (dentistry included).

6 Postgraduate Schools

Although a programmed number of medical students has not yet been approved, access to speciality postgraduate schools is limited. Three facts are worth emphasizing: an ad hoc postgraduate training for general practitioners is still lacking, full-time internship is unusual and a great variety of different speciality schools exists (in 1981, there were more than 140). However, major changes have been made to curricula in recent years, for the purpose of complying with EEC directives and requirements.

In 1981, about 12 000 places were available in all postgraduate medical schools (Table 1), 20% fewer than the 15 000 newly qualified medical students. The provision of these places was sometimes based on available teaching facilities but never on needs or demand criteria. In 1980 (the last year for which data are available), 9336 postgraduate students, i.e. 165 per million inhabitants, obtained a speciality diploma (2).

7 Professional Career

The national distribution of all medical posts occupied is not known. Complete data are provided only for some Regions. Table 2 refers to the Emilia-Romagna Region in northern Italy, with 4 000 000 inhabitants, the capital of which is Bologna. As can be seen, there are 14 332 medical posts in the Region or 3.6 per 1000 population. Of this number, only 47% are directly employed and paid by the INHS, while 53% have contracts, as mentioned earlier. The majority of medical posts are in public hospitals and for general practice. The latter posts are divided into two categories unique to Italy, i.e. community paediatricians, who are paediatric specialists and act as general practitioners for children aged 0–12 years, and community on-call physicians, who are responsible for emergency services at night and during weekends.

The 14 332 medical posts are occupied by 12 400 working physicians, since, as previously indicated, some physicians employed directly by the INHS can also hold a contracted post. In Emilia-Romagna, each physician occupies an average of 1.15 posts (7).

Table 1. Maximum first-year in postgraduate medical schools in 1981 (4). Some minor specialities have been regrouped

Speciality	First-year intake	% total postgraduate posts	Ratio to 1 000 000 population
Anaesthetica (and intensive care)	652	5.6	11.5
Child neuropsychiatry	131	1.1	2.3
Dermatology, dermato-venerology	230	2.0	4.1
Dentistry	460[a]	4.0	8.1[a]
Forensic medicine, criminology	302	2.6	5.3
Internal medicine			
General	348	3.0	6.2
Cardiology	317	2.7	5.6
Chest medicine	411	3.6	7.3
Endocrinology (Diabetology)	293	2.5	5.2
Gastro-enterology	273	2.4	4.8
Geriatrics	181	1.6	3.2
Haematology and Immunology	276	2.4	4.9
Infectious diseases	206	1.8	3.6
Nephrology	73	0.6	1.3
Oncology	205	1.8	3.6
Neurology	301	2.6	5.3
Obstetrics and gynaecology	450	3.9	8.0
Occupational medicine	347	3.0	6.1
Ophthalmology	204	1.8	3.6
Orthopaedics	309	2.7	5.5
Paediatrics and neonatology	741	6.5	13.1
Pathology			
General	380	3.3	6.7
Clinical chemistry	232	2.0	4.1
Microbiology	170	1.5	3.0
Morbid Anatomy	158	1.4	2.8
Nuclear medicine	90	0.8	1.6
Virology	11	0.1	0.2
Pharmacology, toxicology	140	1.2	2.5
Physiotherapy	158	1.4	2.8
Public health (hygiene)	630	5.4	11.1
Psychiatry (see also child neuropsychiatry)	247	2.1	4.4
Psychology	139	1.2	2.5
Radiology	421	3.6	7.4
Statistics	23	0.3	0.4
Surgery			
General and oncological	509	4.4	9.0
Neurosurgery	63	0.5	1.1
Otorhinolargyngology (including audiology)	279	2.4	4.9
Paediatric surgery	55	0.5	1.0
Plastic surgery	44	0.4	0.8
Thoracic surgery – cardiac surgery	153	1.3	2.7
Traumatology	195	1.7	3.4
Vascular surgery	96	0.8	1.7
Other	155	1.3	2.7

Table 1. (continued)

Speciality	First-year intake	% total postgraduate posts	Ratio to 1 000 000 population
Tropical medicine	58	0.5	1.0
Urology	159	1.4	2.8
Others	269	2.3	4.8
Total	11 544	100.0	204.5

[a] 760 first-year students admitted to the new ditistry schools in 1983 must be added to these 460 posts reserved for postgraduate medically qualified students. The overall dentist intakte/population ratio is 21.6 per million.

7.1 Hospital Physicians

Data are available at the national level for hospital physicians. The number of full-time equivalent (FTE)[1] physicians in hospitals tripled between 1961 and 1981, increasing from 4.1 per 10 000 population to 12.1 per 10 000 population (Fig. 5a) The number of hospital beds per physician decreased from 16.5 to 6.4 (Fig. 5b). More recent data are not available; however, the number is likely to have stabilized since all new appointments in the INHS were frozen in 1983.

Hospital physicians working full-time constitute 58% of the total and those working part-time 42%. This proportion of full-time physicians varies among regions, from just over 30% in some southern Regions to more than 80% in a few northern Regions.

The highest densities of public hospital physicians are found in Lazio (Rome) and in Friuli (Trieste) (Fig. 6). Because of variation in the number of beds, the higher number of physicians does not always correspond to a higher physicians/bed ratio, which, however, is not stable. With 10.3 FTE physicians per 10 000 population, Campania (Naples) has fewer beds per physician than Friuli (Trieste), which has 15.5 FTE physicians and 7.3 public hospital beds per physician. Lazio (Rome) has both a high number of public hospital physicians (13.3 per 10 000) and a low ratio of beds per FTE physician (4.7); moreover, Lazio is the Region with the highest proportion of contracted private hospital beds (31% in 1983, as compared with a national average of 16%).

There are three levels for hospital physicians: *assistente*, medical assistant, first level (62% of all public hospital physicians); *aiuto*, assistant chief, second level (23%) and *primario*, chief of service, third and highest level (15%). A law recently passed provides for a new level, that of *assistente in formazione*, assistant in training, but as yet no appointments have been made.

There were 1.9 chiefs of service in public hospitals per 100 000 population in 1981. Over the last few years, the number of posts for hospital physicians at all levels has increased.

---

[1] The number of FTE physicians has been calculated by decreasing by 24% the number of part-time physicians.

Table 2. Frequency distribution of categories of medical posts by number, percentage and ratio to population, Emilia Romagna Region, 1983. The number of medical posts does not coincide with the total number of physicians employed

Category of medical posts by type of appointment	Medical posts No.	%	Rate per 10 000 population
1. Paid directly by INHS			
Public health and occupational medicine	497	3.4	1.3
Community services[a]	487	3.4	1.2
Psychiatry	312	2.2	0.8
Public hospitals	5 393	37.6	13.7
Sub-total	6 689	46.7	16.9
2. Contracted			
General practice	3 638	25.4	9.2
Community on-call service	1 001	7.0	2.5
Community paediatrics	286	2.0	6.3[b]
Out-patient specialists	1 530	10.7	3.9
Contracted private hospitals	1 188	8.3	3.0
Sub-total	7 643	53.3	19.3
General total	14 332	100.0	36.2

[a] Including maternal and child health care.
[b] Per 10 000 children 0–12 years.

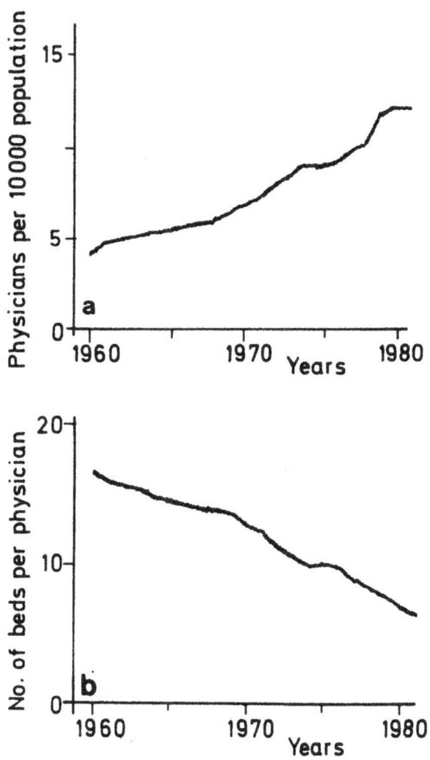

Fig. 5. a FTE public hospital physicians per 10 000 population. **b** Public hospital beds for each physician in the period 1960–1981

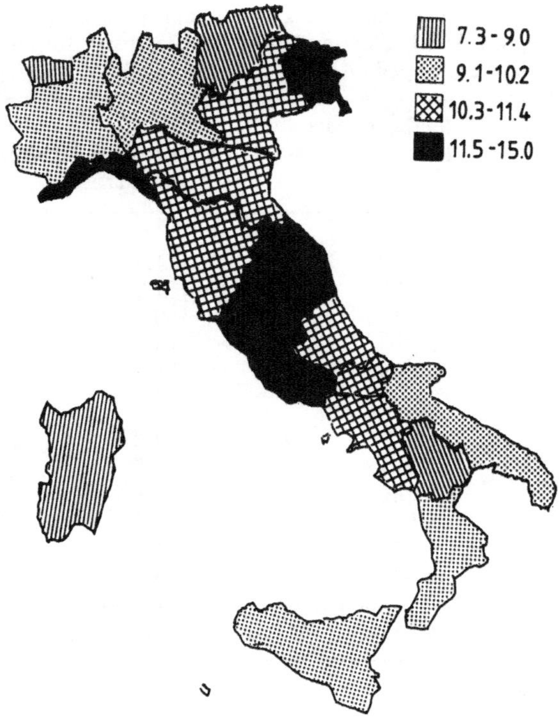

Fig. 6. Distribution of FTE public hospital physicians per 10 000 population by Region, 1981

However, the number of assistants and assistant chiefs increased more than the number of chiefs of service, so that the ratio of level (1 plus 2/3) rose from 4.1 in 1969 to 5.6 in 1981. The ratio of assistants to assistant chiefs has remained stable at about 2.6 to 1. The law mentioned above stipulates a future equalization of the number of assistants and assistant chiefs.

7.2 General Practitioners

As already stated, Italy provides for two roles in primary medical care: general practitioners for adults and community paediatricians for children aged 0–12 years.

The list size cannot exceed the ratio set in 1978, i.e. 1500 adults or 1000 children depending on medical role; however, exceptions are allowed for physicians who had a larger list before 1978.

In 1980 there were 60 026 general practitioners, i.e. 1 per 950 inhabitants, a figure which may vary from 1 per 2500 to 1 per 603 among the various Regions (Table 3). The recommended ratio is 1 : 1000. In that same year, there were few community paediatricians – 1 per 5000 children – because the function of community paediatrician had only recently been introduced and was in competition with private paediatric practice.

Table 3. Distribution of contracted general practitioners by Region, 1980 (8)

Regions	Inhabitants per general practitioner
Piemonte	1394
Valle d'Aosta	1451
Lombardia	1349
Bolzano	2500
Trento	1724
Veneto	1633
Friuli-Venezia Giulia	1426
Liguria	733
Emilia-Romagna	1116
Toscana	938
Umbria	1004
Marche	1266
Lazio	603
Abruzzo	976
Molise	1095
Campania	558
Puglia	1134
Basilicata	1200
Calabria	960
Sicilia	703
Sardegna	1176
Italy	950

The list size distribution is very disparate among the different Regions; in some Regions, more than 40% of general practitioners have fewer than 500 patients while in other Regions more than 40% have over 1500 patients.

7.3 Unemployment and Underemployment of Young Doctors

No official statistics on the number of unemployed physicians are available. However, considering the Emilia-Romagna Region again, a rough estimate of their number can be obtained. For example, in 1983, there were in the Region 17 000 physicians under 70 years of age registered on the Medical Association List. A total of 12 400 physicians were either employed by or contracted to the INHS; however, no fewer than 600, i.e. the 60% of physicians engaged in community on-call services who had only this kind of appointment, may be considered as underemployed. If it is assumed that 7% of registered physicians (mainly dentists) are in private practice only and that 3% do not practise medicine, a rough estimate of 3500 unemployed or underemployed physicians can be obtained, i.e. 20% of the total number of registered physicians under 70 years or almost 1.0 per 1000 population. This estimate supports the often heard but unsubstantiated claim that about 40 000 Italian physicians are unemployed or underemployed.

8 Conclusions

There is undoubtedly an excess of physicians in Italy, and this excess can only increase in the future. If the present trend persists, it has been estimated that there will be more than 400 000 physicians in Italy in the year 2001, 1 per 140 inhabitants or 7.1 per 1000 population (4). However, even if admissions to medical schools were to cease forthwith, there would be about 300 000 Italian physicians in 1991, i.e. 1 per 190 inhabitants or 5.3 per 1000 population.

Many bills have been presented by almost all the political parties for the introduction of desirable programmed numbers of students and for a complete transformation of the medical school curriculum, but none of them has yet been discussed in parliament. There is, however, an acute awareness of the seriousness of this situation.

The updating of the medical curriculum in the past has been essentially additive. Changes to cope with the uncertainties and the new and complex problems facing medicine will have to be made through a complete revision of the study programme.

The number of unemployed or underemployed recent medical graduates is disquieting and constitutes a major obstacle to rational health planning. In particular, any cost-containment policy leads only to saving in monetary rather than human terms if it involves unemployment, underemployment or employment in ineffective activities, and thus a waste of human resources.

The inadequate practical training of many recent medical graduates and the slow development of a suitable autonomous role for nurses are other negative consequences of an inflated medical population. Moreover, the increase in the number of available specialists tends to impoverish the scope of general practice and to increase the general demand for speciality services.

References

1. ISTAT. Annuario Statistico Italiano. Rome, various annual issues
2. ISTAT. Annuario dell'Istruzione. Rome, various annual issues
3. Istituto per la Ricerca di Economia Sanitaria. Disponibilità e fabbisogno di personale medico in Italia al 1985, nel contesto della Comunità Economica Europea. Milan, 1979
4. Magi D, Splendori F, Vanini G (1984) Censimento dei medici italiani al 30 giugno 1984. Suppl al n. 8–9, Anno 3°, Agosto/Settembre 1984, La Rivista Medica Italiana, Rome, 1984
5. Magi D, Parodi E, Poggiolini D (eds) Medici giovani e questione giovanile. Constatazioni dal 1946. Previsioni al 1985. Federazione Nazionale degli Ordini dei Medici. Magi has also published a number of papers for young physicians in search of work in the jounals Il medico giovane and La Rivista Medica Italiana
6. Federazione Nazionale degli Ordini dei Medici. Guida alle Scuole di Specializzazione in medicina e chirurgia. Ragno Editore, Rome
7. Regione Emilia Romagna, Dipartimento Sicurezza Sociale Studi e Programmazione. Relazione Generale sull'attuazione del Piano Sanitario Regional nel triennio 1981–1983. Bologna 1985
8. Consiglio Sanitario Nazionale. Relazione sullo Stato Sanitario del Paese – 1980. Rome, Istituto Poligrafico dello Stato, 1983

United Kingdom

S. Birch and A. Maynard

1 Introduction

The objective of this paper is to appraise critically post-war medical manpower planning in the United Kingdom. Manpower planning should be distinguished at the outset from manpower forecasting. The latter refers to predicting, other things being equal, the future value of a variable, e.g. the future stock of doctors or the future demand for doctors. Planning, on the other hand, is concerned with the manipulation of policy instruments, i.e. other things are not equal over the forecasting period, in order to affect the future stock of doctors. The need for planning arises out of the possibility that future demand will not be met by future supply. Policy decisions by manpower planners are therefore dependent on forecasts of the supply of and demand for future manpower.

It is argued in this paper that there are major weaknesses in the post-war forecasts of both demand for and supply of UK medical manpower and hence in the medical manpower planning conclusions drawn from these forecasts. It is argued further that in order to improve forecasts in the future, the data base on which they are made must be improved. In particular, the present stock of information is deficient in the following areas: (a) data about the characteristics of the population and doctor stock; (b) data about the future changes in the number and characteristics of the population and doctor stock; and (c) data about combinations of medical care inputs to produce a given medical care output.

This paper is divided into four sections. The first section reviews the forecasting of UK medical manpower supply and demand in the post-war period. The second section examines how medical manpower forecasting should be carried out and identifies the data requirements. The third section considers how these data requirements compare with the data currently available. The final section summarises the paper and considers the likely outcome of existing manpower planning policy in the UK.

2 Manpower Forecasting: The UK Experience, 1944–1983

2.1 The Goodenough Committee, 1944

The first attempt to appraise the problems of the market for medical manpower in the post-war period was made by the Inter-Department Committee on Medical Schools under the chairmanship of Sir William Goodenough (1). Its terms of reference were to look into the organization of medical schools in the light of the Government's post-war hospital policy, paying particular attention to the facilities for clinical teaching and research.

The Committee believed that the Government's plans for improvements in health services might necessitate a larger number of doctors in practice than existed at the time. It had no doubt that ".. . . more specialists will be needed . . ." and on the basis of representation from the British Medical Association, it also believed that more general practitioners were needed if they were to provide a " . . . full unhurried service to all patients, to undertake some of the work at present done by public health and school medical officers, to make more regular routine medical examinations and to pay due attention to the maintenance of health as well as the treatment of disease" (page 122). However, the number of general practitioners required would depend upon the form of the future medical service. The Committee therefore doubted whether a useful estimate of the number of additional doctors needed could be made.

The Committee examined how this forecast increase in the demand for doctors would be met by the future supply of doctors. A forecast of doctor supply for the period up to 1963 was provided by the Government Actuary. It was based on the following assumptions: (a) net emigration of doctors would remain at pre-war levels; (b) the wastage rate of medical students would remain at 12.5%; and (c) activity rates would fall in older age groups, i.e. there would be a trend towards earlier retirement. Two alternative sets of age-specific activity rates were used.

On these assumptions, there was the prospect of an increase of several thousands in the civilian doctor stock. Nevertheless, an increase in medical school intake was needed in order to meet the forecasted increase in demand.

The Committee commented on the inadequacies of the published data for accurate manpower planning and recognised that the current data were seriously contaminated by the effects of the war.

The Government accepted one of the main recommendations of the Committee's Report – that greater financial support for medical education was needed – but did not decide on a desirable medical school intake, this being left to individual medical schools to determine independently. During the late 1940s and early 1950s the flow of new doctors emerging from medical schools increased, and by the mid-1950s this was leading to competition for jobs and fears that both jobs and incomes might be adversely affected. These fears, inter alia, led to the appointment of another Committee to examine the problem of medical manpower.

2.2 The Willink Committee, 1957

In response to this increasing competition for consultants' posts in general medicine and general surgery, and for general practice vacancies, a Committee was set up under the chairmanship of Sir Henry Willink to consider the future numbers of medical practitioners and the appropriate intake of medical students (2).

The Committee estimated the demand for and supply of doctors for the period 1956–1971. Forecasted demand was based on the following assumptions:

1. General practice list sizes should be reduced to 2500 on average in non-rural areas and 2000 on average in rural areas (these being arbitrary figures aimed at reducing geographicall inequalities).
2. The total population would increase by 4.5% during the period in question, although the population aged 65 and over would increase by 25% during the same period. This was based on official Government population projections.
3. The age-specific health care demands of the population were based on the estimates of the 1954 Cohen Committee on General Practitioners within the National Health Service (NHS).
4. The service provided by a general practitioner to his patients would remain the same as at that time, i.e. the average number of items per patient per year would remain constant.

5. The number of specialists (i.e. consultants and senior house officers) needed would increase by 160 per annum to 1965 and by 80 per annum thereafter. This assumption was based on a slight reduction in past trends. The Committee estimated that the increased demand for specialists was falling owing to the fact that previously unmet demand was being met and shortages of specialists in rural areas were being removed. However, it was also recognised that expanding medical knowledge, an increasing population and the changing age structure of the population would tend to increase the demand for specialists.
6. The number of junior hospital doctors needed would increase by 700 in order to fill existing vacancies, although this number was reduced in order to take account of the part-time hospital work that would be provided by the increased number of general practitioners. In addition, the demand for junior hospital doctors would increase by the same proportion as the demand for specialists, i.e. the ratio of specialists to junior doctors would remain constant.
7. The demand for doctors employed by local authorities would increase by at least 125 in order to fill existing vacancies.
8. The demand for doctors in academic and research posts would increase by 1% per annum, on the basis of past trends.
9. The additional demand for doctors in industry would fall from 750 at that time, on the basis of existing vacancies, to 280 in 1970–1971.

Overall, the forecast demand for doctors in 1971 was 13% greater than the stock of doctors in 1955. This was compared with the forecasted supply of doctors, which was based on the following assumptions:

1. Retirement rates: past trends of retirement were not suitable as an estimate of future retirement rates, since doctors' activity rates were expected to fall as doctors accrued pension rights under the NHS superannuation scheme. An activity rate of 80% was assumed for doctors under 65. Estimated activity rates of 35% for doctors aged 65 to 70, and of 15% for those aged 70 and over were based on comparisons with other professions, particularly finance, insurance and teaching, where occupational pension rights already existed.
2. Female activity rates: these were assumed to change by the same proportion as those for men.
3. Death rates: age- and sex-specific death rates of the whole population were used as estimates of doctors' future death rates.
4. Part-time work: the proportion of total doctor stock working part-time was assumed to remain constant.
5. Emigration: the number of doctors emigrating would fall once many former colonies had been granted indenpendence and had set up own training facilities.
6. Immigration: the number of doctors from abroad settling permanently in Great Britain would remain the same. The combining of assumption 5. and 6. suggested a net emigration rate of 160 per annum in 1956, decreasing to 50 per annum in 1971.
7. Female students: the proportion of female students would remain at one-fifth of the total.
8. Wastage rates of medical students would remain at 6%.

Comparing the forecasted supply with forecasted demand, the Committe concluded that the present production of new doctors was not too large. The production of doctors in the nex 5 years was predetermined to a large extent by the medical school intake of the previous 5 years. However, the Committee felt that future medical school intake should be cut by 10%. Finally, it suggested that on the basis of a crude estimate of demand beyond 1975, medical school intake should be increased from 1970.

The Government commended the Report to the universities but left the decision on medical school intake to individual medical schools. Within a short period, several of the underlying assumptions of the authors of the Willink Report were subjected to criticism, e.g. Abel-Smith and Gales (3) highlighted the inaccuracy of the Committee's migration assumptions, and comments were made about the weaknesses involved in the use of point estimates for population trends (with no sensitivity analysis).

2.3 The Todd Committee, 1968

In 1965 the Royal Commission on Medical Education was set up under Lord Todd to review medical education in Great Britain " . . . in the light of national needs and resources . . . " (4).

Forecasts of demand were made both for the short term to 1975, for which the production of medical graduates could only be changed by the more intensive use of existing training facilities, and for the long term to the end of the century, for which changes in the provision of training facilities could be considered.

Demand for doctors in 1975 was based in the following targets:

1. The average general practitioner to population ratio for 1961 – 1 : 2180 – should be achieved. This ratio was the lowest recorded up to 1965.
2. The maximum general practitioner list size should be 2500 (2000 in rural areas) in accordance with suggestions of the Ministry of Health.
3. The general practitioner to assistants and trainees ratio should be restored to its lowest recorded figure, i.e. that for the period 1953–1955.
4. The hospital doctor targets for 1968 set by the Regional Hospital Board reviews, following the report of the Platt Committee on Medical Staffing Structure in the Health Service, should be achieved. The 1968 targets were adjusted for the expected increase in population for the period 1968–1975.
5. There should be an expansion of demand for doctors to work overseas, on the basis of reports of the Ministry of Overseas Development.
6. There should be an expansion of the number of doctors employed in Britain outside the hospital services and general practice in proportion to the expansion in population.

The targets in 1.–4. and 6. were applied to estimates of the population in 1975. This was based on an average annual increase of 0.8% derived from forecasts of the Registrar General. This estimate implied that the proportion of the population over 65 would rise slightly, while the proportion in the 45–54 cohort would fall. The effect which varying of this age distribution would have on demand was predicted to be slight. The reason for this is that the effect produced by varying the birth rate assumptions affects total population estimates, but the effect on the demand for services is less great since the major users of health services are the elderly and their numbers are not affected in the short term by different assumptions concerning birth rates. Hence the need for medical services was taken to vary directly with the projected total population size.

When all these factors were taken together, the resulting doctor to population ratio estimated for 1975 was observed to be greater than that for 1965 by an amount equal to an annual increase of 1.25%. This was consistent with observations of the change in the ratio throughout the century. In terms of doctor numbers, it suggested that 78 100 economically active doctors would be required by 1975, an increase of 16 600 over the 1965 figure.

Turning to the predictions of long-term demand, the Committee felt unable to incorporate the uncertainty of future developments into a specific forecast. In particular, uncertainty surrounding changes in the pattern of medical care, the future population and the effect of changing standards of living on expectations of medical care led the Committee to present a broad picture of what future demand might be. This was based on an extrapolation of the past trend of an average annual increase in the doctor per population ratio of 1.25%. However, it was suggested that additional pressures for more time spent in training and leisure would require an annual increase greater than this. Moreover, the changing age structure of the population would lead to changes in the relative need for health services.

Using Swedish data on the relative costs of care for the old and the young to weight the population, the Committee predicted a reduction in medical care requirements per unit of the population as a result of the increasing proportion of the population under 40. It suggested that an annual increase of 1.5% in the doctor per population ratio might be sufficient to satisfy the additional pressure discussed above. After weighting for the changing age structure of the population, this would give an annual increase of 1.3% in the ratio. The Committee suggested that this would be consistent with resource constraints based on the following assumptions: (a) an average annual increase in national income of 3%; (b) a constant proportion of national income spent on health serives; and (c) a reduction in the increased real expenditure on the health services of 1.5% owing to the real price effect.

This gives rise to a total of 119 800 doctors required by 1995. The Committee did stress, however, that this prediction was sensitive to the population projection and should be reassessed in the light of changes in this projected figure.

The Committee's forecast of the future supply of doctors was based on the existing number of doctors, with changes to this stock estimated through use of the following assumptions:

1. New medical graduates: the output of medical schools for the next five years was predetermined by medical school intake of the previous 5 years. Current planned intake figures for the following 5 years were used. A wastage factor of 10% was applied to medical school intake, based on observed wastage rates of recent years. The proportion of new medical graduates that would be female would remain constant.
2. Deaths: age- and sex-specific death rates for the whole of England and Wales were applied to the forecasted doctor stock to estimate losses due to deaths. This assumed that (a) death rates would not change over the next ten years and (b) that doctors experienced the same death rates as the population as a whole.

The Committe recognised that (b) was not strictly correct but argued that the differential between general and doctor death rates was small and the conclusions were not sensitive to this assumption.

3. Activity rates: the projected activity rates of the Willink Committee were used after adjustment for the forecast increase in the proportion of younger women doctors at work. No allowance was made, however, for a change in the contribution of women doctors overall to medical practice, i.e. the proportion of women among doctors in active practice was assumed to remain at 16%.
4. Emigration: forecasts of net emigration were based on recent experience and observed trends. The results of a study by Abel-Smith and Gales (3) of a 5% sample of doctors for the period 1925–1959 formed the basis of the estimate. Immigration from less developed countries was considered separately. This was seen as being demand-determined to a large extent, and an estimate of future immigration of this type was based on what could reasonably be demanded of these countries in terms of the supply of qualified doctors. The estimated figure for net emigration was 180 per annum, decreasing to 100 per annum from 1975 to 1980, with zero net emigration thereafter.

The Committee concluded on the basis of these forecasts that there would be a deficit of 10 000 doctors over the next 10 years, and proposed three possible courses of action: (a) the introduction of new medical schools; (b) the reorganization of existing medical schools; and (c) more intensive use of existing medical schools as currently organised.

The report of the Committee accepted however that " . . . much of the statistical information which would form the basis of [the calculation of exact requirements] is lacking . . ." (page 284).

The Government accepted the recommendation for immediate expansion increasing the targeted medical school intake to 1975. However, a decision on the longer-term recommendations of the Report was deferred.

2.4 The Royal Commission on the National Health Service, 1979

In 1976 a Royal Commission was set up under Sir Alec Marrison to consider " . . . the best use and management of the financial and manpower resources of the National Health Service" (5).

Although the Commission recognised that the number of doctors which the United Kingdom should train was clearly of great concern, it did not feel able to conduct a major review of the manpower situation with the time available. However, a study (6) of the supply of doctors up to the year 2000 was commissioned " . . . to stimulated and inform public discussion of the issues".

The authors of the study – Maynard and Walker – made a number of forecasts of the future supply of doctors to the year 2000, based on different assumed values of certain variables. The assumptions common to all the forecasts were:

1. Mortality rates were assumed to remain the same throughout the period, and foreign-born doctors were assumed to experience the same death rates as British-born doctors.
2. Losses of medical graduates to non-NHS fields of medicine were assumed to be 1% per annum.

3. Activity rates for males were assumed to be those predicted by the Todd Report, with the additional assumption that all doctors would retire at 70 if they had not already done so.
4. The age distribution of new entrants to the doctor stock was assumed to be the same for both sexes.
5. The current emigration rate of foreign-born doctors was taken as an estimate of the future emigration rate of this category.

The variables for which alternative values were considered were:

1. Sex and nationality composition of the new medical graduates, for which three different compositions were considered
2. Migration rates of British and Irish doctors, for which three sets of values were considered
3. Immigration rates of foreign (non-Irish) doctors, for which three sets of values were considered
4. Female participation rates, for which two sets of values were considered

The authors considered in detail three combinations of these assumptions: a "best guess" based on their own intuitions of "best guess", the lowest forecast and the highest forecast. The results of the forecasts in terms of the predicted doctor stock in the year 2000 were 89 765, 72 134 and 98 606 respectively.

Maynard and Walker then considered the resource implications of the alternative forecasts, noting that the changing numbers and age structure of the medical profession have implications for the relative numbers in general practice, hospital practice and community medicine, and consequently the resource requirements of the NHS. The commented (page 26):

> Whilst it may be easy to commit society to more doctors by emotive and imprecise arguments and the use of crude time series ratios showing greater numerical availability of such personnel, the resource consequences in terms of other goods and services foregone, should not be ignored. More doctors means more expenditure on medical training, medical salaries and medical expenditure (in hospitals and in primary care). Such activities consume resources which are scarce and which could perhaps be used to greater advantage elsewhere in our community.

On the basis of the report and on evidence provided by different sections of the medical profession, the Commission thought that the planned output of medical graduates was about right and that medical unemployment was unlikely before the end of the century.

2.5 Medical Manpower – The Next Twenty Years, a Government Discussion Paper (1978)

In 1978 the Government published a discussion paper concerning medical manpower planning for the next 20 years (7). The purpose of the paper was to consider whether changes in medical student intake were required in order to meet the future demand for doctors. The paper did not make a single forecast of the number of doctors required by the end of the century but made estimates of the number of extra doctors that would be needed if specific targets were to be reached. In particular, it considered the effect on doctor demand of:

1. Maintaining the 1975 doctor to population ratio
2. Bringing all regions up to the 1977 average level of hospital staffing
3. Eliminating designated areas (those with a high average population per general practitioner ratio) by reducing their average ratio to 2500
4. Reducing contracted hours of junior doctors to 80 hours per week and of consultants to 40 hours per week
5. Reducing the average ratio of population per general practitioner to 2100
6. Ensuring desirable growth, as specified in other reports, in various shortage specialities
7. Increases in community medicine
8. Increases in the academical medical staff

Various factors which would affect doctor demand were not considered owing to the difficulty in quantifying them, e.g. changes in the proportion of various grades, effects of technological change, improvements in services, demands for specialists in occupational medicine and growth in the private sector.

It was not suggested that these demands could or should be met, but the forecasts were intended "to give a series of possible choices for using an increased number of doctors . . .". The sensitivity of the forecasts to the estimates of the future population was recognised, and upper and lower estimates of future fertility rates were used in arriving at the forecasts. However, a major assumption underlying the forecasts was that the pattern of delivery of medical care was to remain unchanged and that the role of the doctor would be as much as it was in 1976.

In order to put the forecasts of demand in perspective, an estimate was made of the change in the amount of resources that might be devoted to health service provision. Alternative assumptions of the growth of gross national product (GNP) – of 3% and 2.5% – were made. It was assumed that the proportion of GNP devoted to the health services would not change and that the real price effect would reduce the real growth of resources by 1.5% per annum. It was further assumed that the proportion of health service resources devoted to employing doctors would remain the same. This would depend on the change in doctors' salaries relative to other health service costs and the mode of delivery of health care. However, the number of doctors in the hospital service was observed to have grown in line with the real costs of the service in the previous 15 years.

These assumptions led to the forecasts that an annual increase of 1.5% (or 1.0% on the basis of 2.5% growth rate in GNP per annum) could be supported. This forecasted expansion in demand is increased to 2% if the proportion of resources devoted to health services were to grow by 1% over the next 20 years.

It was suggested therefore that a figure of between 1% and 2% should be taken as the annual increase in demand for doctors for the purpose of medical manpower policy. It was stressed, however, that the forecast should be reconsidered in the light of the debate concerning the assumptions underlying this estimate.

Whilst awaiting response to the discussion paper, the Government set up a Steering Group called upon, as stated in its report (8), "to co-ordinate studies of supply of and demand for medical manpower in relation to the likely availability of resources up to the end of the century" (page 1).

In view of the fact that the demand for health services would be "virtually unlimited in the absence of financial constraints" (page 6), attention was focused on the possible developments of NHS expenditure over the next 20 years. On the assumption of (a) an annual growth in gross domestic product of 2% per annum; (b) an increase in the share of expenditure of health and personal social services, the basis of evidence from other countries as national income grows; (c) a relative price effect which would reduce the increase in real expenditure on health services to something between 1.5% and 2% per annum; and (d) a continuation of the present mode of delivery of health services, an overall growth rate in the demand for doctors of between 1% and 2% was forecasted. The alternative forecasts depended on assumptions about (a) whether the number of doctors would grow at the same rate as expenditure or faster than expenditure, as previously observed and (b) whether hospital and community health current expenditure were to grow at 1% per annum (the minimum to keep pace with demographic change), 1.4% per annum (a figure suggested to Regional Health Authorities in 1978 as a resource assumption in preparing plans to 1989), or a more optimistic figure of 2% per annum.

The forecasted supply of doctor manpower made in the 1978 discussion paper (DHSS 1978) was based on the following assumptions:

1. Contracted hours of consultants and junior hospital doctors would be reduced to 40 and 80 hours per week respectively.
2. The target medical school intake of 4080, once achieved, would be maintained.
3. The proportion of the medical school intake born abroad would remain constant.
4. The proportion of the medical school intake that is female would increase to 50%.
5. The wastage rate of medical students would be the same as in the previous few years.
6. There would be a net emigration of 0.6% of doctor stock.
7. A total of 25% of doctors over 65 would be active at the beginning of the forecast period, this figure decreasing to 12% at the end.
8. Women doctors would be active for 36 years on average (27 years' whole-time equivalent) at the beginning of the period, this number rising to 39 on average (30 years' whole-time equivalent) at the end.

Separate forecasts of doctor supply were made by the Steering Group for differing assumptions for 6. and 7. above.

The main conclusion of the analysis was that on the basis of the projections made, present policies concerning medical manpower would not result in massive over-production of doctors. Three short-term problems, however, were forecast:

1. The number of pre-registration posts would need to be increased in line with the forecasted increase in medical graduates from 3000 to 3600.
2. The ratio of career posts to training posts had to change to accomodate the increasing proportion of doctors seeking permanent employment. Cutting the number of graduates in order to match the present career openings would solve the problem only if the hospital service could be run with substantially fewer doctors overall than at that time.
3. The problem of "shortage specialities" was likely to remain.

The Steering Group's report confirmed these findings, concluding that the available information "does not provide grounds either for departing from the present medical school target intake or for altering it once it has been reached" (page 49). However, the uncertainties surrounding the projections were recognised, and regular updated calculations based on the most comprehensive information available were recommended.

Other recommendations made were for increasing flexibility in the career structure in order to respond to unanticipated changes in any of the variables affecting demand for doctor, and for more information to be provided on the possibilities of labour substitution.

2.6 An Overview of the UK Experiences

What is clear from that above is that forecasting the demand for doctors has been generally rather ad hoc. The British tradition has been to extrapolate trends, using time series data on doctor-population ratios, and then to add to this estimates of demand for "shortage specialities", for instance, geriatrics and mental handicap, make an allowance for the reduced working hours of doctors and include a forecast for the reduced list size for general practitioners (see [9] and [10] for further discussion of this). All these ad hoc calculations can be queried. The time trends require analysis rather than casual and unthinking adoption for extrapolation purposes. The doctor-population ratio is a crude aggregate index which fails to take account of the varying contributions of different sections of the doctor stock on the one hand the varying needs of the different sections of the population on the other. Both the denominator and the numerator in this ratio need weighting for these differential characteristics of the heterogenous groups they are intended to represent.

General practitioners may or may not provide better care if they have smaller numbers of patients for whom to care. Similarly, doctor inputs in mental handicap may be queried, cure is not possible and care may be best provided by other inputs (e.g. clinical psychologists). Forecasts have failed to separate the demand for health care from the demand for doctor and hence have assumed, either explicitly or implicitly, that the mode of delivery of health care is to remain unchanged. Issues such as these can be elaborated but have unfortunately not been resolved.

Despite these problems, the tradition has been to use such crude methods and to determine, usually, casually, whether their resource implications could be met. Generally, these estimates were crudely produced and not subjected to much sensitivity analysis.

The predictions of the Goodenough Committee were based on general practitioners' allowing more time per patient and spending part of their time in other fields of medicine, without consideration being given to whether such time would be productive in terms of health outputs and, moreover, to whether it was more efficient to provide such services through general practitioners or other medical personnel. Little attention was paid to the resource implications of the findings.

The Willink Committee's forecasts of demand for doctors were based on extrapolations of part trends. As such, they were subject to the same weaknesses as those of the Goodenough Committee. Indeed, both emigration and immigration were seriously underestimated by the Committee, and as a result, by 1965 there were substantially more doctors in Britain, although fewer British-born doctors, than had been predicted. Futhermore, the Willink Committee used the official population projections of the mid-1950s, which proved to have substantially underestimated the increase in population in the early 1960s. Again, the forecasts of the Committee were not considered in the light of forecasted future resources.

The Todd Committee's forecasts of demand for doctors were based on extrapolations of the existing crude doctor-population ratio added to estimates of existing "unmet need" in shortage specialities. The weakness of this methodology has been discussed above, but the Committee's conclusions were further contaminated by overestimates of the population increase in the forecast period.

Neither the Willink Committee nor the Todd Committee considered the sensitivity of its predictions to its population projections, despite the fact that estimates of the future population size must be about as uncertain as any other variable in the forecasting of doctor demand.

The 1978 discussion paper (7) did recognise the problems outlined above. It noted that individual elements of the doctor stock making up the total differed markedly and, similarly, that the population should be weighted to take account of the differing needs of cohorts of the population. Recognition was given to the role of the doctor as just one input of the health production process and to the fact that estimates of doctor demand would be sensitive to the relative importance of the doctor in this production process, the evolution of other social services, the changing disease patterns in society and the future availability of resources. Once these considerations have been introduced, a "more modest approach" to demand estimation is then adopted, one which assumes that most of these variables will remain constant in the future and proceeds to forecast future demand by using targets of doctor-population ratios within predicted future resource constraints. This is done because of the lack of information and uncertainty surrounding these other factors. Similarly, the Steering Group's report (8) based its demand estimations on forecasts of future resource constraints.

The methodology adopted for estimating the future supply of doctors has tended to be on much firmer ground. The existing stock of doctors is measured and estimates of future changes in this stock are made. Where the forecasts of future supply have been suspect is in the assumptions used for estimating the changes in the doctor stock.

Forecasts of supply of doctors would be affected by errors of two main types. First, there is the failure to recognize the importance of a particular variable in the supply of doctors. For example, the Goodenough Committee did not consider the effect of a change in the proportion of females among new medical graduates on the supply of doctors. The failure to recognize such an effect is equivalent to assuming that the variable is to remain constant throughout the forecast period. Second, the importance of a variable in doctor supply may be recognized, but the estimate of its value may be wrong. For example, the Willink Committee underestimated the rate of increase in the number of hospital doctors.

Summarising the importance of demand forecasts' being resource-based (i.e. costed in the light of alternative assumptions about the growth of resources in the forecasting period) appears to have become accepted in recent manpower planning exercises. A second point, however, which has not entered official forecasts to date is that over the forecasting period "other things may not be equal". This applies equally to forecasts of demand and supply.

3 Forecasting Medical Manpower – The Way Forward

3.1 Demand

Forecasting the demand for doctors should begin with the basic question "Why are doctors in demand?" The answer is that doctors are in demand because they combine with other inputs of labour and capital to produce health services which, it is hoped, lead to improvements in health. The demand for doctors is therefore dependent on the demand for health services, i.e. it is a derived demand. The first stage in forecasting demand must therefore be to decide on the priorities, e.g. what forms of health improvements are to be provided first and to what extent. Hence, the mere fact that general practice lists exceed a total of 2000 patients each should not in itself be a matter of concern. Only if a reduction in the size of general practice lists increased the output of health care and this improvement were felt desirable over and above all other improvements in health care that could be achieved by using the same resources should a reduction in the size of general practice lists be considered a priority. Such a process of policy formation leads to the identification of a set of policy targets; which should then be considered in relation to the resources avaialable, i.e. the budget constraint must be determined.

The next step is to consider the alternative means of attaining these policy targets. For example, what are the alternative combinations of doctors and nurses to a hospital ward for mentally handicapped patients? A major weakness of existing forecasts of the demand for doctors has been their assumption of ceteris paribus conditions over the forecasting period, i.e. they assume that the mode of delivery of health care is to remain the same. No attemps have been made to appraise product mixes, e.g. the best mix of nurses, doctors, drugs and capital to care for patients in a particular client group, and possibilities for input substitution in the production of health care. This assumption of fixed input coefficients in the production of health care has prevented the identification of different and potentially more efficient means of achieving the policy targets.

The demand for inputs, including all types of labour inputs (i.e. manpower), can then be derived from the identified efficient means of reaching specified targets. A further implication of the possibilities of input substitution is that the demand for one type of input, e.g. doctors, is dependent on the demand for other inputs. Hence, the planning of different types of medical manpower is interdependent.

3.2 Supply

The future supply of doctors is estimated by taking the existing stock of doctors and amending this figure on the basis of a forecasted net increase in the doctor stock. These changes in doctor stock depend on a number of factors, e.g. the output of new medical graduates, net doctor emigration, death and retirement of doctors, etc. This then gives a forecast of the total number of doctors in the future. The output of health care from a given doctor stock, however, depends inter alia on the composition of that stock. For example, the work of doctors in training is different from that of fully trained doctors, and the activity rate of doctors may differe between the sexes. Consequently, forecasting the supply of doctors should involve estimating not only the size of the doctor stock but also its characteristics.

A second point to note is that the outpout of health care from a given doctor stock also depends on the availability of other health care inputs. However, this does not affect the manpower planning for doctors, provided that the demand size forecasting procedure has been followed through as above, since (a) alternative forms of provision of health care would have been considered and appraised, and (b) planning of all forms of medical manpower would be performed simultaneously, with the result that bottlenecks in the production of health care should not occur.

When the future demands for and supply of doctors, as well as other health care inputs presumably, have been considered, the forecasts can be compared in order to determine how policy must be manipulated to achieve balances between supply and demand in all input markets.

All the stages of this procedure must be repeated with various underlying assumptions being used in order to consider the effects of changes in assumptions on the forecasts, i.e. sensitivity analysis, and hence on the policy conclusions. This sensitivity analysis can be complemented with calculations about the resource implications of the alternative forecasts. Furthermore, these procedures should be repeated at regular intervals (e.g. biannually) in order to incorporate developments accruing during the elapsed period and hence rendering some of the alternative assumptions redundant and others more pertinent.

3.3 Information Requirements of Good Manpower Forecasting

What are the data requirements of these desirable procedures? The first requirement is an accurate and readily accessible data base describing the existing situation. This is not merely concerned with the exact number of doctors and accurate figures on the size of the population. It was shown above that the data base must also include information on all the characteristics of the population and the doctor stock which affect the demand for and supply of health care.

Second, the procedures require the appropriate information on which to base forecasts of the future number and characteristics of both the population and the doctor stock. Extrapolation of past trends is alone insufficient unless it can be substantiated by existing evidence. Information may already be available to suggest that the future value of a variable will not be a continuation of a past trend. Forecasting the future necessarily involves a considerable degree of uncertainty, but this uncertainty can be reduced by incorporating as much relevant information as possible. Futhermore, the uncertainty can be recognised explicitly by performing sensitivity analysis on the forecasts, using the highest and lowest possible values of the variables whose future values are uncertain.

Third, information is required on the alternative means of producing the desired health care objectives, i.e. the different combinations of inputs that may be used to produce the desired medical output.

4 Medical Manpower in the 1980s – The Strengths and Weaknesses of the Data

In this section we consider to what extent the published information and data satisfy the demands of good manpower forecasting as decribed in the previous section. In doing this we examine the current supply of doctors in the UK from a stock and flow perspective.

4.1 The Demand for Medical Manpower

4.1.1 Statements of Policy Targets

The Department of Health and Social Security (DHSS) has from time to time considered the priorities for future health services. For example, consultative documents were published in 1976 and 1977 (11, 12) which set target rates of growth for the various services. Priority was given to the future expansion of services for the elderly and mentally handicapped. These targets, however, were framed in terms of the Government's published plans for public expenditure on health and social services, which extended only to the fiscal year 1979–1980. With regard to long-term planning of medical manpower demand, policy targets are not stated, but expected demand is based on past trends, forecasted changes in the demographic structure of the population and arbitrary reductions in the population-doctor ratios. This lack of a clear statement on long-term policy targets tends to encourage resource allocation within the health care sector by incremental budgeting, i.e. competing programmes tend to have the same priority as in the previous period and hence are allocated the same amount of resources as before, with marginal changes in relative priorities restricted to the distribution of any increase in the total real resources devoted to the health care sector. There is therefore a need for more information on the long-term policy targets of the health care sector.

4.1.2 Population Projections

Information is required on the size and nature of the future population in order to consider the resource implications of the policy targets. Population projections for the next 40 years are published annually by the Office of Population Censuses and Surveys (e.g. 1980 [13]). The projections are calculated by applying age- and sex-specific death rates, age- and sex-specific migration rates and age-specific fertility rates to the estimated mid-year population estimate of the base year. The assumptions on which the present projections are based are: (a) age-specific mortality rates will decrease by a constant proportion each year on the basis of past trends; (b) the age/sex structure of different streams of emigrants and immigrants is based largely on past trends; (c) alternative assumptions concerning fertility are made, thus providing a range of population projections; and (d) recent trends in marriage and divorce rates will continue in the immediate future and then level out.

The population projections are categorised according to age, sex and marital status and reported for England and Wales, Wales, Scotland and Great Britain on the basis of the "principal projection", i.e. that projection based on an assumed fertility rate just sufficient to maintain the native population without taking account of the effects of emigration and immigration ("replacement level fertility"). The differences in the age- (but not sex-) specific population are recorded for the alternative assumptions of high and low birth variants.

Existing forecasts have noted that although alternative assumptions concerning fertility affect the numbers in this group is the set of future age- and sex-specific mortality rates. power is small. This is because the major consumers of health care are the elderly, whose numbers are already known for the period of the forecast. However, one factor that does affect the numbers in this group is the set of future age- and sex-specific mortality reates. In order to take account of the uncertainty surrounding future mortality rates in relation to the future demand for medical manpower, sensitivity analysis should be performed on the population projections with respect to mortality rates.

The resulting population projections are reported by age, sex and marital status. However, no account is taken of birthplace, which may be an important determinant of the health care needs of individuals. Furthermore, the population projections are not recorded according to region, other than the broad regional classifications of England, Scotland and Wales.

Briefly, the major weaknesses of the data on population projections are that (a) sensitivity analysis is not performed for alternative assumptions about future death rates, although variations in this variable are those which have the greatest effect on future health care demands; (b) the data are not categorised by origin or ethnic group; and (c) the data are not categorised by region.

4.1.3 Forecasted Resource Constraints

Information about the planned expenditure on health care is restricted to the period of the next 4 years, as published in the Government's annual White Paper on Public Expenditure. Long-term forecasts of demand must therefore be based on assumptions concerning (a) the future level of national income and (b) the proportion of national income to be devoted to health care in the future.

Neither of these variables can be predicted with any confidence for any period other than that of the immediate future. For example, the gross domestic product increased by less than 6% over the period 1974–1981 (14), as compared with estimates of between 2.5% and 3% per annum used in the forecasts. Nevertheless, forecasts for future demand must consider future resource constraints, and attempts to estimate this constraint must avoid the crude extrapolation of past trends of either of the above-mentioned variables unless there are good reasons why past trends should continue.

4.1.4 Alternative Means of Producing Health Care

There has been relatively little systematic analysis of alternative forms of production of health care, although research in North America suggests that the opportunities for substitution among different medical care inputs are considerable (15, 16). The importance of information on substitution of inputs is in determining the most efficient, i.e. least expensive, way of producing a given health care output. However, even if substitution possibilities can be identified, an additional problem is to change the providers' behaviour in order to adopt the most efficient means of production.

At present, increasing the efficiency of medical practice often brings little reward to the doctor, i.e. the person ultimately responsible for the delivery of health care. Hence, even when substitution possibilities are identified, there is no incentive for the doctor to take advantage of the efficiency gains arising out of their implementation (for further discussion of incentives in the persuit of efficiency in health care delivery see [13]. Information on input substitution possibilities is therefore of no use unless there is reason to believe that substitution of inputs is likely to be made by those individuals responsible for delivery of medical care.

To summarize, if forecasting of the demand for medical manpower is to be improved, the following information should be provided:

1. Information on the long-term service targets of the health care sector
2. Information on the future population, by birthplace and region
3. Information on the sensitivity of the population projections to different assumptions concerning mortality rates
4. Information on the possibilities of input substitution, which, to be of use to manpower forecasts, should be backed up by incentives to those responsible for the delivery of health care to use the most efficient form of production of health care.

4.2 The Supply of Doctor Manpower

4.2.1 The Existing Stock of Doctors

Information on the existing stock of doctors is published annually by the DHSS in the case of England (17), by the Scottish Home and Health Department, for Scotland (18) and by the Welsh Office (19), for Wales (data for England alone are reported below). These data on doctors are reported according to the following categories:

1. The sector of the Health Service in which they are employed, i.e. as hospital staff, community health staff or general practitioners, in number or whole-time equivalents (WTEs) (Table 1). There is a certain overlap of categories, since some doctors recorded under the community health service also appear elsewhere in the data. The DHSS does correct for the double counting, but the corrected data are not generally published. It can be seen from Table 1 that there were 36 476 hospital doctors and 24 359 general practitioners in England in 1981. During the period 1974–1981, the hospital doctor stock grew by 24.5% and the general practitioner stock by 13.1%.
2. The region in which they work measured in WTEs and WTE per 100 000 population (Tables 2 and 3). The distribution of general practitioners is recorded separately, while the data for hospital and community health staff are included in a single category, that of directly employed medical and dental staff. Separate categories for hospital and community health doctors are not recorded in the published data. The data in Table 3 show that the geographical distribution of hospital doctors and general practi-

Table 1. Medical manpower 1974–1981 at 30. September. (From [17])

	Unit	England					
		1974	1977	1978	1979	1980	1981
Directly employed medical staff							
Total[a]	WTEs	29 293	32 653	33 490	34 578	35 759	36 476
of which							
Hospital medical staff		26 946	29 909	30 692	31 768	32 924	33 579
Community medical staff		2 347	2 744	2 799	2 810	2 835	2 897
General medical practitioners							
Total[b]	No.	21 531	22 327	22 651	23 062	23 674	24 359
of which							
Unrestricted principals		20 219	20 796	21 040	21 357	21 812	22 304
Restricted principals		313	290	271	251	233	214
Assistants		464	375	343	311	276	280
Trainees		535	866	997	1 143	1 353	1 561

a Excludes hospitals practitioners, part-time medical officers (clinical assistants), general medical practitioners participating in Hospital Staff Funds and occasional sessional staff in community health services for whom no WTE is collected.

b Figures relate to 1 October.

tioners in England was very uneven in 1980, ranging from 69.9 to 98.6 per 100 000 population for the former category and from 47.6 to 57.1 per 100 000 population for the latter.

Each of these categories of employment is then recorded separately by various categories:

A Hospital Medical Staff

1. By grade, sex and nature of contract of employment, i.e. whole-time, part-time or honorary staff measured in numbers and WTEs (Tables 4 and 5). The data in Table 4 show that the number of doctors increased by 24% in the period 1974–1981 and that the number of consultants and senior hospital medical officers increased by 17% during the same period. However, the proportions of female doctor stock and female consultants increased from 8% to 16% and from 2% to 11%, respectively, during the same period. The data in Table 5 show that the substantial increase in female participation in the period under review is spread across all grades and for both full-time and part-time work. The number of full-time female doctors has increased by 61% and the number working part-time by 45%. In the case of consultants and senior hospital medical officers the corresponding growth rates are 86% and 29%.
2. By grade and age, measured in numbers (Table 6). The data in Table 6 show the changing age structure of the total doctor stock and the stock of consultants and senior hospital medical officers. Over the 4-year period 1978–1981, the proportion of these stocks under 40 years old rose from 63% to 65% and from 19% to 21%, respectively, while the proportion over 60 years old fell from 5.5% to 4.5% and from 13.5% to 11%, respectively.
3. By speciality and grade (Tables 7 and 8). The data in Table 7 show that the "shortage specialities", e.g. geriatric medicine and mental illness, expanded much faster during the 7-year period 1974–1981 – by 53% and 33% respectively – than the more popular specialities, e.g. general surgery, whose growth over the same period was 11%. Table 8 shows that these patterns are not restricted to one grade of speciality.
4. By grade and place of birth (Table 9). The data in Table 9 show the reduction in the proportion of overseas-born doctors in the stock of hospital doctors, from 34.9% in 1974 to 31.4% in 1981. However, the opposite trend is observed in the stock of consultants and senior hospital medical officers, an increasing proportion of the stock – 16.9% in 1981, as compared with 13.9% in 1974 – having been born abroad. This can probably be explained by the reduction in doctor immigration during the period in question and hence by a lower proportion of overseas-born doctors entering the sub-consultancy grades. This effect has not had time to filter through to the proportion of consultants born overseas.

B General Practitioners

1. By type (Table 10). General practitioners are allocated to one of four categories:
   a) Unrestricted principal: a practitioner who provides the full range of general medical services and whose list is not limited to any particular group of persons
   b) Restricted principal: a practitioner who provides either the full range of general medical services to a restricted population (e.g. the staff of one or more hospitals

Table 2. Medical manpower by region at 30 September 1980[a]. (From [17]) WTEs Number[b]

	England	Northern	Yorkshire	Trent	East Anglian	North West Thames	North East Thames
Directly employed medical and dental staff[c]	38 217	2513	2568	3183	1332	3381	3541
General medical practitioners[a, b]	23 674	1493	1784	2169	957	1957	1937

a General medical practitioner figures relate to 1 October.
b Numbers of practitioners are included; other figures are WTEs.
c Figures exclude hospital practitioners, part-time medical or dental officers, clinical assistants, general practitioners participating in Hospital Staff Funds and occasional sessional staff in community health services for whom no WTE is collected.

Table 3. Medical manpower by region (per 100 000 population) at 30 September 1980. (From [17]), WTEs per 100 000 population[a]

	England	Northern	Yorkshire	Trent	East Anglian	North West Thames	North East Thames
Directly employed medical and dental staff[b]	82.2	81.5	71.7	69.9	70.8	98.6	95.6
General medical practitioners	50.9	48.4	49.8	47.6	50.9	57.1	52.4

a For medical and dental staff and all practitioners, mid-1980 home population figures have been used in the calculation of these ratios; for all other staff, the populations used take account of the populations served by the regions rather than of the populations living within their boundaries.
b Excludes hospital practitioners, part-time medical or dental officers, clinical assistants, general practitioners participating in Hospital Staff Funds and occasional sessional staff in community health services from whom no WTE is collected.

South East Thames	South West Thames	Wessex	Oxford	South Western	West Midlands	Mersey	North Western	London postgraduate teaching hospitals
3293	2380	1859	1707	2249	3778	2006	3456	971
1863	1545	1386	1140	1743	2501	1218	1981	–

South East Thames	South West Thames	Wessex	Oxford	South Western	West Midlands	Mersey	North Western
92.8	83.3	68.8	74.0	69.7	73.3	82.0	86.3
52.5	54.1	51.3	49.4	54.1	48.5	49.8	49.5

Table 4. Medical manpower in hospitals: by total and by specialist grade, 1974–1981 (at 30 September). (From [17])

	England											
	1974		1977		1978		1979		1980		1981	
Grade and sex	No.	WTE	No.	WTE	No.	WTE	No.	WTE	No.	WTE	No.	WTE
All staff (excluding hospital practitioners and paragraph 94 appointments)												
Total	27 576	25 618	30 520	28 397	31 515	29 293	32 607	30 356	33 475	31 431	34 218	32 142
Male	23 169	21 643	25 023	23 405	25 657	23 966	26 263	24 569	26 789	25 331	27 160	25 681
Female	4 407	3 975	5 497	4 992	5 858	5 328	6 344	5 786	6 686	6 101	7 058	6 461
of which, consultant's and senior hospital medical officers with allowance												
Total	10 623	9 373	11 382	10 124	11 640	10 382	11 891	10 632	12 134	11 090	12 397	11 347
Male	9 728	8 608	10 288	9 180	10 450	9 349	10 613	9 515	10 784	9 897	10 975	10 098
Female	895	765	1 094	944	1 190	1 033	1 278	1 117	1 350	1 193	1 422	1 249

or similar institutions) or maternity medical services and/or contraceptive services only

c) Assistant: a practitioner who acts as an assistant to a principal

d) Trainee: a practitioner employed for a maximum period of 1 year for the purposes of training in general practice and in respect of whom a training grant is paid.

The data in Table 10 show the trend away from smaller practices towards larger partnerships. In 1969, 23% of unrestricted principals operated single-handed, compared to 27% operating partnerships of three of more. The corresponding figures for 1981 are 13% and 45%, respectively. The data also show the increasing number of trainees. This is due to the introduction of the 3-year post-registration training for general practitioners, 1 year of which is spent as a general practitioner trainee to an existing principal. There appears to have been some substitution of trainee time for assistants whose numbers have declined over the same period.

2. By age and sex (Table 11). The data in Table 11 show an increase in the proportion of female general practitioners from 12% in 1969 to 18% in 1981. In the context of a 20% increase in the total number of general practitioners during this period, this means that the number of female general practitioners increased by 86% between 1969 and 1983. The data also show a change in the age structure of the stock of general practitioners, with the proportion under 40 rising from 28.5% in 1969 to 37% in 1981, whilst the proportion aged 60 and above fell from 14% to 13% over the same period.
3. Unrestricted principals by place of birth (Table 12). The data show that the stock of unrestricted principals has become increasingly dependent on doctors born overseas, the proportion having risen from 13.8% in 1969 to 22.3% in 1981.
4. Unrestricted principals by region, measured in number of principals and average list size (Table 13). Although the range of average list size by region has fallen, the average list size of the worst-served region in 1981 (Trent, 2309) was still 12.5% greater than the best-served region (South Western, 2053). Furthermore, the relative positions of the regions were very similar throughout the period 1974–1981.
5. Other grades by region (Table 14). These data are measured in terms of the number of practitioners, without being related to the population served, and interpretation of the regional differentials is therefore difficult.

C. Community Health Medical Staff

Community health medical staff have less direct contract with patients but are more involved in planning and evaluating health service options. The data in Table 15 show that this sector grew by 34% in terms of the numbers employed over the period 1974–1981, although in terms of WTEs the growth was more modest (23%). This sector provides a good opportunity for part-time work, a fact which is no doubt responsible for the large (and increasing) proportion of females employed in community medicine.

There are some differences in categorisations between the date for England and Wales and those for Scotland. Details of these differences will be provided in a subsequent draft.

Table 5. Medical manpower in hospitals: by total, by specialists and by contract, 1974 and 1981 (at 30. September). (From [17])

	1974						
	All staff		Whole-time staff	Part-time staff		Honorary staff	
	No.	WTE	No.	No.	WTE	No.	WTE
All staff (excluding hospital practitioners and paragraph 94 appointments)							
Total	27 576	25 618	19 853	6 249	5 057	1 474	708
Male	23 169	21 643	16 484	5 344	4 515	1 341	644
Female	4 407	3 975	3 369	905	542	133	63
of which consultants or senior hospital medical officers with allowance							
Total	10 623	9 373	4 133	5 473	4 717	1 017	523
Male	9 728	8 608	3 743	5 039	4 379	946	487
Female	895	765	390	434	339	71	36

4.2.2 Factors Affecting the Future Supply of Medical Services

There are a numer of factors which affect the future stock of doctors and the supply of medical services from this stock.

4.2.2.1 The Production of New Medical Graduates

In the UK the undergraduate education of a doctor takes 5 years, i.e. essentially 2 years of basic science and 3 years of clinical work. Graduation is followed by 1 year (the pre-registration year) of study, consisting of 6 months of medicine and 6 months of survery. The doctor is then registered with the General Medical Council. Normally, training as a hospital specialist requires a further 6 years of post-registration training, although progression through the training grades to a consultancy post may take much longer. The Royal Colleges arrange in-training examinations and set qualifying arrangements which have to be met prior to examination. The acquisition of Royal College qualifications seems to be essential for career progression in some specialities, e.g. general surgery or general medicine.

Since 1981, all new general practitioners have had to undergo 3 years of post-registration training, consisting of 2 years of hospital work and 1 year of attachment as a trainee to a general practitioner who is a principal. Table 16 gives details of the number of students admitted to medical schools and the number obtaining medical degrees in Great Britain in the academic year 1981–1982. These data are collected by the University Grants Committeee (UGC).

1981						
All staff		Whole-time staff	Part-time staff		Honorary staff	
No.	WTE	No.	No.	WTE	No.	WTE
34 218	32 142	25 237	6 513	5 630	2 468	1 277
37 160	25 681	19 806	5 198	4 761	2 156	1 117
7 058	6 461	5 431	1 315	870	312	160
12 397	11 347	5 559	5 466	5 055	1 372	736
10 975	10 098	4 831	4 905	4 602	1 239	667
1 422	1 249	728	561	453	133	69

Medical school intake has been increasing steadily towards the Government's target of 4080 annually by the mid-1980s. An additional factor to be noted, however, is that the proportion of women entering and graduating from medical school continues to increase (43% and 37%, respectively, in 1981–1982).

The number of students graduating from medical school depends on the wastage factor, i.e. the number dropping out of school or failing. Crude wastage rates based on the proportion of entrants not gaining a qualification within 5 years fail to take into account the varying lengths of medical courses and interruptions in 5-year courses. In the 1978 discussion paper (7), the following effective wastage rates were calculated on the basis of new qualifiers in the period 1965–1972 to take into acount those factors:

	GB-born	Irish-born	Overseas-born
Male	8.4%	20%	22%
Female	6.5%	20%	20%

Although such figures are not calculated and published on a regular basis, the Department of Education and Science publishes data annually on the numbers of medical students in each year of the various medical courses. The decreasing proportion of students on 6-year courses does imply that crude wastage rates should be falling, ceteris paribus, as more students qualify to register within 5 years of commencing undergraduate studies.

Table 6. Medical manpower in hospitals, by total and by specialists by age 1978–1981 (at 30 September). (From [17])

Grade		England All ages	Under 30	30–34	35–39	40–49	50–59	60–64	65 and over	No. Age not known
All staff (excluding hospital practitioners and paragraph 94 appointments)										
Total	1978	31 515	9 140	6 730	4 214	5 555	4 140	1 570	159	7
	1979	32 607	9 595	6 838	4 541	5 745	4 232	1 444	190	22
	1980	33 475	10 030	6 965	4 679	5 931	4 240	1 472	158	–
	1981	34 218	10 565	6 852	4 901	6 037	4 255	1 438	170	–
Consultants and senior hospital medical officers with allowance	1978	11 640	4	522	1 738	4 221	3 595	1 437	123	–
	1979	11 891	5	522	1 825	4 389	3 674	1 324	152	–
	1980	12 134	3	564	1 901	4 550	3 659	1 336	121	–
	1981	12 397	1	581	2 027	4 668	3 679	1 302	139	–

Table 7. Medical manpower in hospitals: by speciality, 1974–1981 (at 30 September). (From [17])

Speciality	Unit	England 1974	1977	1978	1979	1980	1981
All specialities:	No.	27 576	30 520	31 515	32 607	33 475	34 218
total	WTE	25 617	28 397	29 292	30 356	31 431	32 141
of which:							
General medicine	No.	3 662	3 934	4 130	4 196	4 246	4 277
	WTE	3 398	3 667	3 846	3 920	3 988	4 018
Anaesthetics	No.	2 979	3 322	3 445	3 572	3 644	3 747
	WTE	2 792	3 147	3 254	3 384	3 491	3 597
General surgery	No.	3 182	3 300	3 400	3 474	3 501	3 532
	WTE	3 042	3 142	3 232	3 315	3 378	3 410
Mental illness	No.	2 317	2 652	2 732	2 824	2 962	3 087
	WTE	2 158	2 459	2 543	2 624	2 755	2 871
Obstetrics and	No.	2 198	2 333	2 354	2 381	2 422	2 475
gynaecology	WTE	2 061	2 196	2 216	2 243	2 313	2 358
Orthopaedic	No.	1 542	1 651	1 712	1 776	1 815	1 845
surgery	WTE	1 476	1 582	1 648	1 712	1 759	1 796
Paediatrics	No.	1 281	1 461	1 512	1 609	1 692	1 829
	WTE	1 185	1 336	1 390	1 485	1 569	1 690
Geriatric medicine	No.	944	1 190	1 239	1 360	1 419	1 453
	WTE	914	1 154	1 212	1 328	1 387	1 422
Accident and	No.	974	1 173	1 212	1 274	1 342	1 381
emergency	WTE	966	1 165	1 199	1 262	1 333	1 372
Radiology	No.	987	1 062	1 110	1 163	1 223	1 253
	WTE	932	1 001	1 049	1 102	1 172	1 205

Staff holding hospital practitioner and paragraph 94 appointments are not included in this table.

Table 8. Medical manpower in hospitals: by speciality and grade, 1974 and 1981 (at 30 September). (From [17])

		England			
		1974		1981	
Speciality		All staff	Consultants and senior hospital medical officers	All staff	Consultants and senior hospital medical officers
All specialities	No.	27 576	10 623	34 218	12 397
	WTE	25 617	9 373	32 141	11 347
of which					
General medicine	No.	3 662	980	4 277	1 088
	WTE	3 398	823	4 018	959
Anaesthetics	No.	2 979	1 361	3 747	1 598
	WTE	2 792	1 239	3 597	1 528
General surgery	No.	3 182	888	3 532	895
	WTE	3 042	778	3 410	836
Mental illness	No.	2 317	933	3 087	1 119
	WTE	2 158	837	2 871	1 010
Obstetrics and gynaecology	No.	2 198	628	2 475	674
	WTE	2 061	547	2 358	626
Orthopaedic surgery	No.	1 542	559	1 845	629
	WTE	1 476	506	1 796	597
Paediatrics	No.	1 281	370	1 815	498
	WTE	1 185	325	1 679	447
Geriatric medicine	No.	944	277	1 453	399
	WTE	914	269	1 422	391
Accident and emergency	No.	974	78	1 381	122
	WTE	966	77	1 372	121
Radiology	No.	987	668	1 253	804
	WTE	932	624	1 205	774

Staff holding hospital practitioner and paragraph 94 appointments are not included in this table.

Table 9. Medical manpower in hospitals: by grade and place of birth, 1974–1981 (at 30 September). (From [17])

Grade and place of birth	England 1974 No.	%	1977 No.	%	1978 No.	%	1979 No.	%	1980 No.	%	1981 No.	%
All staff												
All places of birth	27 576	100.0	30 520	100.0	31 515	100.0	32 607	100.0	33 475	100.0	34 218	100.0
UK or Irish Republic	17 949	65.1	20 236	66.3	20 984	66.6	21 856	67.0	22 715	67.9	23 472	68.6
Elsewhere	9 627	34.9	10 284	33.7	10 531	33.4	10 751	33.0	10 760	32.1	10 746	31.4
Consultant and senior hospital medical officers allowance												
All places of birth	10 623	100.0	11 382	100.0	11 640	100.0	11 891	100.0	12 134	100.0	12 397	100.0
UK or Irish Republic	9 144	86.1	9 659	84.9	9 811	84.3	9 989	84.0	10 134	83.5	10 300	83.1
Elsewhere	1 479	13.9	1 723	15.1	1 829	15.7	1 902	16.0	2 000	16.5	2 097	16.9

Staff holding hospital practitioners and paragraph 94 appointments are not included in this table.

Table 10. General medical practitioners by type of practitioner, 1969–1981 (at 1 October). (From [17])

	England 1969	1977	1978	1979	1980	No. 1981
All practitioners						
Total:	20 208	22 327	22 651	23 062	23 674	24 359
Unrestricted principals						
Total	18 901	20 796	21 040	21 357	21 812	22 304
Single handed	4 131	3 419	3 335	3 179	3 089	2 990
Partnerships of 2	4 828	4 198	4 134	4 054	4 016	4 004
Partnerships of 3	4 875	4 917	4 968	5 096	5 112	5 132
Partnerships of more than 3	5 064	8 262	8 599	9 028	9 595	10 178
Restricted principals	495	290	271	251	233	214
Assistants	641	375	343	311	276	280
Trainees	171	866	997	1 143	1 353	1 561

Table 11. General medical practitioners by age and sex, 1969–1981 (at 1 October). (From [17])

		England 1969	1977	1978	1979	1980	No. 1981
All ages	Total	20 208	22 327	22 651	23 062	23 674	24 359
	Male	17 820	18 836	18 971	19 197	19 525	19 912
	Female	2 388	3 491	3 680	3 865	4 149	4 447
Under 30		966	1 612	1 629	1 758	1 843	1 941
30–39		4 809	5 546	5 855	6 219	6 681	7 168
40–49		6 657	6 100	6 039	5 953	6 012	6 077
50–59		4 848	5 870	6 016	6 123	6 065	6 059
60–64		1 477	1 828	1 753	1 636	1 668	1 692
65–69		931	734	742	782	828	833
70 and over		520	637	617	591	577	589

Unrestricted principals, restricted principals, assistants and trainees included.

Table 12. General medical practitioners: unrestricted principals by place of birth, 1969–1981 (at 1 October). (From [17])

	England 1969		1977		1978		1979		1980		1981	
	No.	%	No.	%	No.	%	No.	%	No.	%	No.	%
All places of birth Total	18 901	100.0	20 796	100.0	21 040	100.0	21 357	100.0	21 812	100.0	22 304	100.0
Great Britain Total	14 584	77.1	15 417	74 1	15 575	74.0	15 736	73.7	15 980	73.3	16 258	72.9
Other UK or Irish Republic Total	1 732	9.1	1 289	6.2	1 209	5.8	1 135	5.3	1 095	5.0	1 068	4.8
Elsewhere Total	2 585	13.8	4 090	19.7	4 256	20.2	4 486	21.0	4 737	21.7	4 978	22.3

Table 13. General medical practitioners: Unrestricted principals by region, 1974–1981 (at 1 October). (From [17])

Region	England 1974	1977	1978	1979	1980	1981
England: Total						
No. of principals	20 219	20 796	21 404	21 357	21 812	22 304
Average list size	2 384	2 331	2 312	2 286	2 247	2 201
Northern						
No. of principals	1 301	1 339	1 357	1 376	1 400	1 432
Average list size	2 471	2 399	2 377	2 342	2 291	2 237
Yorkshire						
No. of principals	1 515	1 574	1 593	1 620	1 658	1 694
Average list size	2 422	2 342	2 318	2 285	2 235	2 186
Trent						
No. of principals	1 833	1 926	1 943	1 973	2 021	2 054
Average list size	2 527	2 428	2 419	2 385	2 342	2 309
East Anglian						
No. of principals	766	805	830	858	871	894
Average list size	2 282	2 257	2 214	2 175	2 163	2 118
North West Thames						
No. of principals	1 691	1 717	1 724	1 739	1 779	1 820
Average list size	2 305	2 267	2 266	2 263	2 233	2 194
North East Thames						
No. of principals	1 731	1 727	1 742	1 741	1 779	1 803
Average list size	2 354	2 320	2 299	2 299	2 258	2 221
South East Thames						
No. of Principals	1 620	1 656	1 663	1 685	1 714	1 740
Average list size	2 365	2 294	2 282	2 256	2 232	2 197
South West Thames						
No. of principals	1 323	1 353	1 347	1 365	1 407	1 420
Average list size	2 288	2 275	2 302	2 284	2 229	2 215
Wessex						
No. of principals	1 136	1 205	1 225	1 245	1 272	1 325
Average list size	2 308	2 233	2 217	2 201	2 170	2 102
Oxford						
No. of principals	927	976	1 004	1 027	1 063	1 095
Average list size	2 411	2 368	2 334	2 316	2 268	2 221
South-Western						
No. of principals	1 469	1 499	1 529	1 552	1 581	1 623
Average list size	2 170	2 169	2 140	2 128	2 102	2 053
West Midlands						
No. of principals	2 171	2 226	2 251	2 300	2 336	2 395
Average list size	2 447	2 394	2 371	2 325	2 293	2 233
Mersey						
No. of principals	1 045	1 070	1 090	1 116	1 131	1 158
Average list size	2 466	2 400	2 358	2 301	2 257	2 210
North-Western						
No. of principals	1 691	1 723	1 742	1 760	1 800	1 851
Average list size	2 465	2 415	2 377	2 347	2 297	2 234

4.2.2.2 Career Choices of New Medical Graduates

The DHSS publishes information annually (see [20]) on medical staffing prospects in the NHS by speciality in order to help new medical graduates in choosing the speciality in which they wish to practice. The information consists of:

1. Details of doctor numbers in each speciality by grade and sex
2. Details concerning consultants' post advertised in the previous 12 months by speciality, as follow:
   a) Number of posts becoming vacant
   b) Number of posts unfilled
   c) Number of candidates per post
   d) Percentages of successful candidates (1) female and (2) trained overseas
   e) Previous grades of successful candidates
   f) Mean number of years which the successful candidates spent at the grade immediately below, i.e. senior registrar level
   g) Mean age of successful candidates when this is first post at this grade
3. Details concerning senior registrars' post advertising in the previous twelve months by speciality, as in 2. above
4. Expected annual retirements of consultants, by speciality, for the next 10 years, based on existing retirement patterns
5. Average annual growth in the number of consultants' posts for the past 5 years, by speciality

In contrast to this information on expected future opportunities, Parkhouse et al. (21) survey annually the career preferences of newly qualified doctors. The first 7 years covered by these surveys have been summarised below in oder to consider trends in career preferences.

The overall career preferences of the seven cohorts of qualifying doctors were found to be similar. A comparison of these preferences with the opportunities within the NHS suggests that general practice and community medicine are not attracting the interest of enough qualifiers, despite the information provided by the DHSS described above. Analysing the preferences by sex reveals no significant change over the 7 years. However, the increasing proportion of female graduates and the increasing activity rates of female doctors suggest that those specialities which tend to be favoured more by women, e.g. ophthalmology, accident and emergency, and community medicine, might be expected to increase in popularity.

It could be argued that the preferences revealed by female doctors are determined by the nature of the speciality, e.g. as regards the ability to follow the speciality whilst raising a family. The increasing activity rate of female doctors should not alter these relative preferences; indeed, if anything, we might expect them to be strengthened since the increase in the number of female doctors in practice has been matched by an even greater increase in the number of female doctors practising part-time, i.e. part-time appointments are becoming even more important to female doctors (see section on activity rates below).

4.2.2.3 Doctor Immigration

Doctors wishing to practice in Breat Britain who qualified abroad must register with the General Medical Council (GMC). There are three categories of registration open to doctors who qualified abroad:

Table 14. General medical practitioners by type and region, 1 October 1981. (From [17])

	England						
	England	Northern	Yorkshire	Trent	East Anglian	North West Thames	North East Thames
All practitioners	24 359	1537	1823	2214	996	2020	1970
Unrestricted principals	22 304	1432	1694	2054	894	1820	1803
Average list size	2 201	2237	2186	2309	2118	2194	2221
Restricted principals	214	8	6	8	9	33	29
Assistants	280	12	18	16	15	49	21
Trainees	1 561	85	105	135	78	118	117

1. Full registration: this entitles a doctor to engage in any form of professional employment. The doctor must be of good character, have the necessary knowledge of English to practise medicine in the UK (see below), hold a medical qualification recognised by the GMC and have completed 1 year's satisfactory service as a resident house officer in the UK or have equivalent experience.
2. Provisional registration: this entitles the doctor to work only in resident posts in hospitals approved for the purpose of pre-registration service. The requirements for provisional registration are as for full registration, with the exception of the 1 year's service as a resident house officer.
3. Limited registration: this is normally granted only for supervised employment in hospitals approved by one of the Royal Colleges for educational and training purposes. The period for which limited registration is granted may not exceed a total of 5 years. The requirements for this category of registration are much the same as for provisional registration, with the exception that many overseas qualifications acceptable for limited registration would not be acceptable for provisional registration.

The regulations do not apply to qualified doctors of the member states of the EEC who are eligible for full registration.

Data are not generally published on doctor immigration, although the DHSS is able to derive figures on the annual inflow of doctors into Great Britain from the Central Medical Research Council (CMRC). These data are usually classified by place of birth as opposed to place of training. The 1978 discussion paper published provisional figures on the annual inflow of doctors for the per 1962–1975. These are produced in Table 17. Furthermore, an age distribution of the inflow by sex and place of birth was calculated on the basis of the average values for the period 1965–1972. These are reproduced in Table 18.

Limited information is available about trends in deaths, emigration and activity reates of these doctors. The GMC publishes annual details of new registrations and the numbers

							No.
South East Thames	South West Thames	Wessex	Oxford	South-Western	West Mid-lands	Mersey	North Western
1897	1564	1462	1184	1788	2588	1270	2047
1740	1420	1325	1095	1623	2395	1158	1851
2197	2215	2102	2221	2053	2233	2210	2234
20	22	7	7	13	22	13	17
24	28	9	16	27	18	10	17
113	94	121	66	125	153	89	162

ceasing to be registered, for both provisional and full registration. This information is not suitable for estimating doctor immigration, however, since it does not include details for limited registrations. Furthermore, it pertains strictly to registration and not to doctor movements. A doctor may register without even being resident in Great Britain, provided that the registration requirements are met.

As far as future levels of immigration are concerned, there have been a number of changes in recent years which might affect the inflow of doctors. The 1978 Medical Act withdrew recognition, for full registration purposes, of the qualifications of certain countries and changed the criteria for full registration. The Professional and Linguistics Board (previously the Temporara Registration Assessment Board) tests attempts to control the quality of immigration doctors (of the 1420 candidates sitting the test in 1976, only 506 (36%) passed). Changes in the emigration regulations of some countries have also been made. These factors will either discourage overseas doctors from seeking employment in Great Britain or reduce the number available because they cannot meet the new criteria.

On the other hand, doctors not qualified for full registration may be eligible for limited registration, from which it will be possible to progress to full registration. However, there is a 5-year maximum period of limited registrations, whereas temporary registration (the predecessor of limited registration) could be renewed for an unlimited period of time.

Finally, implementation of the EEC directives on the free movement of labour might lead to increased doctor immigration from the EEC Member States. At present, data are not published separately for doctors from EEC countries. Data on GMC registrations show that the number of EEC doctors with full registration increased from 183 in 1979 to 364 in 1982. However, doctor registrations do not necessarily correspond with doctor stock, as was noted above. Clearly, more information is needed on doctor immigration in order to make useful forecasts of future doctor stocks.

Table 15. Community health manpower by grade and sex, 1974–1981 (at 30 September). (From [17])

	England											
	1974		1977		1978		1979		1980		1981	
Grade	No.	WTE	No.	WTE	No.	WTE	No.	WTE	No.	WTE	No.	WTE
All staff[a]												
Total	4509	2347	5655	2734	5835	2782	5885	2795	5981	2821	6035	2883
Male	2155	1054	2611	1117	2674	1108	2670	1088	2702	1096	2721	1118
Female	2354	1294	3044	1617	3161	1674	3215	1707	3279	1725	3314	1765
Community medicine staff												
Total	515	513	810	766	785	736	790	737	798	733	808	739
Male	389	388	569	533	563	522	556	512	557	506	551	500
Female	126	125	241	234	222	214	234	225	241	227	257	239
Clinical medical staff												
Total	3994	1835	4845	1968	5050	2047	5095	2057	5183	2088	5227	2144
Male	1766	666	2042	585	2111	586	2114	575	2145	590	2170	618
Female	2228	1169	2803	1383	2939	1460	2981	1482	3038	1498	3057	1526

[a] Excludes occasional staff.

Table 16. Number of students admitted to pre-clinical courses and number obtaining a first registrable qualification, Great Britain 1981–1982. (Source: UGC personal communication

	Total	Male	Female
Admissions	3919	2240	1679
Qualifying	3387	2124	1263

Table 17. Immigration into Great Britain of fully or provisionally registered doctors, by place of birth. (From [7])

	Born in UK or Irish Republic	Born outside UK and Irish Republic
1962–1964	1090	2390
1964–1965	530	1630
1965–1966	560	1940
1966–1967	580	1870
1967–1968	590	2100
1968–1969	520	2100
1969–1970	650	1630
1970–1971	530	1450
1971–1972	700	1730
1972–1973	670	1850
1973–1974	560	1800
1974–1975	570	1470
1975–1976		
1976–1977		
1977–1978		
1978–1979		
1979–1980		
1980–1981		
1981–1982		
1982–1983		

4.2.2.4 Doctor Emigration

Data concerning doctor emigration are as scarce as for doctor immigration. The DHSS is able to derive data from the CMRC on the annual outflow of doctors from Great Britain, and those for the period 1962–1975 are reproduced in Table 19.

What is evident from the data in Table 19 is that no clear trend exists in doctor emigration. This ought to be expected since emigration will depend not only on opportunities for doctors in Great Britain but also on opportunities abroad. There is no reason why these should be consistently related.

The trend in the 1970s was for countries (e.g. United States, Canada, Australia and New Zealand) which had previously been popular destinations for emigrant British doctors to restrict doctor immigration. On the other hand, new opportunities for overseas work have arisen with the implementation of EEC directives on the free movement of labour within

Table 18. Age distribution of inflow into Great Britain: analysis by age, sex and place of birth. (From [7]). Percentage inflow in given age band

	Place of birth					
	Northern Ireland		Irish Republic		Elsewhere	
Age	Male	Female	Male	Female	Male	Female
Under 25	0	0	0	0	0	0
25–29	24	43	54	46	42	49
30–34	36	23	18	12	34	28
35–39	15	11	8	13	13	12
40–44	9	11	7	13	5	5
45–49	5	5	5	6	3	3
50–54	4	2	4	5	1	1
55–59	3	1	2	2	1	1
60–64	2	1	1	1	1	1
65–69	1	1	1	2	0	0
70–74	1	1	0	0	0	0
75 +	0	1	0	0	0	0

Table 19. Emigration from Great Britain of fully or provisionally registered doctors, by place of birth. (From [17])

	Born in UK or Irish Republic	Born outside UK and Irish Republic
1962–1964	1640	2050
1964–1965	1050	1260
1965–1966	940	1070
1966–1967	1030	1390
1967–1968	1070	1360
1968–1969	840	900
1969–1970	940	1250
1970–1971	860	1530
1971–1972	810	1330
1972–1973	1040	1230
1973–1974	1010	1170
1974–1975	1040	1020
1975–1976		
1976–1977		
1977–1978		
1978–1979		
1979–1980		
1980–1981		
1981–1982		
1982–1983		

Member States. More information is needed on how these changing opportunities have affected doctor emigration from Britain.

The Medical Register is of little help in estimating doctor emigration, since it only records doctor registrations not doctor movements. An emigrant doctor may continue his registration whilst practising abroad. Furthermore, removals from the register are classified according to know death, removal at doctor's own request, non-reply to registration correspondence or non-payment of registration fees. None of these categories are of use in identifying emigrant doctors.

The DHSS considered the age and sex structure of the emigrants. The data presented in Table 20 are derived from the CMRC and are based on average rates for the period 1965–1972. No information is available on trends in these figures, and no details are published on the grade, speciality, region or sector of employment of the emigrants. Many of these doctors may return to practise in Great Britain at a later date; however, they would then be included in the doctor immigration of UK-born doctors (see Table 17).

Much more information on the characteristics of emigrant doctors is needed in order to make accurate forecasts of the size and characteristics of the future doctor stock.

4.2.2.5 Deaths

There is no generally published information on the number of deaths of doctors. Although the GMC records the numbers of members ceasing to be registered because of death, it may be that many members ceasing registration for other reasons (e.g. non-payment of fees, non-reply to correspondence) are also dead. The 1978 discussion paper reported age- and sex-specific death rates for doctors, based on the average rates for the period 1965–1972 as derived from the CMRC. These are reported in Table 21.

No information is given as to whether these rates differ according to speciality, region, place of birth or training. Previous manpower forecasts have used age- and sex-specific mortality rates for the whole population as estimates of future mortality rates of doctors.

Table 20. Emigrant doctors by age, sex and place of birth (annual flow per 10 000 stock at given age). (From [7])

Birthplace	Great Britain		Northern Ireland		Irish Republic		Elsewhere	
Age	Male	Female	Male	Female	Male	Female	Male	Female
Under 25	–	–	–	–	–	–	–	–
25–29	332	375	660	1160	1040	860	740	680
30–34	385	263	1510	1030	1140	710	1340	1070
35–39	227	169	970	240	760	500	1380	980
40–44	124	79	170	200	290	280	870	520
45–49	79	76	90	150	160	200	460	270
50–54	51	48	60	120	110	160	220	160
55–59	41	39	50	110	90	150	140	60
60–64	46	44	60	120	100	160	90	80
65–69	50	44	70	130	120	180	80	40
70–74	25	26	60	80	110	120	60	50
75 +	25	26	50	40	90	60	60	20

Table 21. Death rates: analysis by sex (deaths per year per 10 000 in stock at a given age). (From [7])

Age	Males	Females
Under 25	6	6
25–29	8	7
30–34	11	9
35–39	15	12
40–44	23	17
45–49	39	25
50–54	66	37
55–59	107	56
60–64	182	91
65–69	330	152
70–74	1195	282
75 +	2011	661

The 1978 discussion paper (7) noted that the death rates calculated were very close to those for social class 1 as a whole. Hence, estimates of future mortality rates might be based on estimates of this groups mortality rate unless there are a priori reasons for believing that this pattern will change in the future. Official Government population projections assume mortality rates will decline in the future along a trend line observed in the past. However, there is no theoretical foundation for that assumption.

There is clearly a need for information on the number and characteristics of death rates amongst doctors.

4.2.2.6 Activity Rates

So far, consideration has been given to the number, and changes in the number, of doctors. The variable that links these data will the supply of medical services is the activity rates of the doctor stock. As with most of the categories discussed above, data on doctors' activity rates are not generally published. Should activity rates of doctors differ by any particular characteristic, e.g. age, sex, place of birth, etc., the calculation of the supply of medical services will be sensitive to assumptions on activity rates.

The 1978 discussion paper (7) provided information by age, sex and place of birth on the percentage of the doctor stock active in medical practice in 1974. The data were derived from the CMRC and are reproduced in Table 22.

As far as trends in doctor activity rates are concerned, the discussion paper (7) noted that the activity rates of doctors under 65 appeared to be rising (mainly owing to the increased activity of 60–65 year olds), while those of doctors over 65 were falling. It appears that retirement ages are becoming less variable for male doctors as a whole and are concentrating around the age of 65. In Britain, most hospital doctors have to retire at 65, but there is no retirement age for general practitioners.

The DHSS publishes data each year on the expected annual number of retirements from consultancy posts in the next 10 years, by speciality. These data are based on the assumption that existing retirement patterns will continue in the future; hence, over a period of

Table 22. Activity rates: analysis by age, sex and place of birth (percentage of stock at given age active in medicine in 1974). (From [7])

Age	Males			Females		
	Great Britain	Ireland	Elsewhere	Great Britain	Ireland	Elsewhere
Under 25	100	100	100	100	100	100
25–29	100	100	100	97	99	99
30–34	100	100	100	89	97	96
35–39	99	99	99	89	95	94
40–44	99	99	99	90	93	93
45–49	99	99	99	90	91	92
50–54	99	99	98	89	91	91
55–59	98	98	98	85	92	87
50–64	91	94	95	69	82	82
65–69	51	56	64	29	49	51
70–74	24	34	32	13	21	22
75 +	9	19	21	6	8	9

time they will change as (a) the age structure of the consultant stock changes and (b) existing retirement patterns change. The data relate only to consultants' posts, and no information is given on the regional distribution of the expected retirements.

In the case of women, recent studies by Ward (22) and Day (23) suggest that the number of female doctors not practising medicine has fallen considerably but that at the same time, the proportion of women doctors practising part-time has risen. When both these factors are taken into account, the contribution of women doctors to medical care appears

Table 23. Part-time working (percentage of active stock working part-time at age shown). (From [7])

Age	Males	Females
Under 25	4	(6)
25–29	3	27
30–34	2	39
35–39	3	47
40–44	5	44
45–49	6	48
50–54	7	44
55–59	7	(45)
60–64	16	(46)
65–69	48	(72)
70–74	(54)	(77)
75 +	(67)	(100)

In cases where the sample analysed contained fewer than 100 doctors of the specified sex in a given age band, the percentage is bracketed.

to be increasing. This information is of even more importance once it is applied to the data on the proportion of medical graduates who are female.

Figures on part-time working are not generally published. However, the 1978 discussion paper (7) considered data based on a 10% sample of the 1971 census. The figures reproduced in Table 23 must be treated with caution since the numbers of doctors of given age groups were, in most cases, small.

5 Concluding Overview

5.1 The Current Balance

The 1980 Steering Group Report (8) concluded that the existing production of doctors in the UK is "about right" in order to meet estimated demand to the end of the century. We will consider the assumptions on which the forecasts, and hence the conclusion, were based.

5.1.1 Forecasts of Demand

1. An average annual rate of increase in gross domestic product (GDP) of 2% would appear to be over-optimistic on the basis of the prevailing economic climate and observed growth rates for 1974–1981.
2. There is no reason to believe that the share of public expenditure on health and personal social services will rise continually either on the basis of continued growth of GDP or on the ground that the share of public expenditure on health is positively correlated with GDP. Indeed, the present Government is pledged to cut public expenditure, and this must inevitably put pressure on the share of funds allocated to the NHS.
3. A continuation of the present mode of delivery of health care would appear to be a conservative assumption.

It is not suggested that accurate estimates of alternative values of the variables can be made. The impartant point is that for each of these assumptions, the expected error leads to an overestimate of the demand for doctors, while lower rates of economic growth, less public expenditure and the substitution of other inputs for doctors must inevitably put downward pressure on doctors' income and employment levels in the next decade.

5.1.2 Forecasts of Supply

1. The proportion of medical students born abroad may fall owing to the substantial increase in undergraduate fees in recent years.
2. The target of a medical school female intake of 50% appears unlikely to be met by 1985.
3. Death rates for doctors are less than those for the population as a whole.

4. General practitioners still appear unwilling to retire at 65, despite the fact that it was expected in the Willink Report and subsequent reports that they would do so.
5. Emigration is unlikely to rise because of the "oversupply" of doctors in the EEC countries, North America and Australia.

5.2 Implications for the Future

It appears that if the assumptions made turn out to be wrong, the direction of the error is likely to favour there being "to many" as opposed to "too few" doctors available in the UK. This will lead to doctor unemployment and/or lower salaries, as was forecast by Maynard and Walker (9).

This pessimistic conclusion is not mitigated by Government attempts to increase the consultant to junior doctor ratio in the NHS hospital sector, as recommended by the Short Committee (24). This recommendation arose out of the recognition that the ratio of consultants to junior doctors will fall as the increasing output of medical schools replaces the reduced immigration of doctors, who in the main are not looking for careers in the NHS and hence are not seeking consultants' posts. The recommended increase in the number of consultants' posts would allow for this structural shift (and a reduction in contracted hours of junior doctors to a maximum of 80 hours a week).

Members of the Government argue that fully trained doctors would produce a better quality and greater quantity of services which would be reflected in the faster throughput of hospital patients, reduced out-patient attendances and fewer diagnostic tests (25). It is therefore argued that the increased salary bill of such a structural shift would be offset to a large degree by these "efficiency" gains.

Such an argument, however, fails to recognize many implications of the proposed structural shift:

1. No evidence has been produced to support the assumption that fully trained doctors are more efficient in providing health care.
2. Increasing the number of consultants would increase the demand for other health care inputs. Newly appointed consultants would not see themselves as performing the same duties as junior hospital doctors. Hence, if there were more consultants, there would naturally be more theatres, secretarial services, etc.
3. With more consultants, there may be a problem over the division of labour. With fewer juniors to carry out routine procedures, consultants would be obliged to fill the gap. Who would decide the distribution of work-loads among the specialists and according to which criteria?
4. Even if efficiency gains were achieved as assumed, this would result in a larger number of patients being treated, i.e. costs per patient would fall, but total costs would rise as more patients were treated.

The logical conclusion to be drawn from the recommendation to increase the ratio of consultants to junior doctors is that there would be a significant increase in total costs above the planned growth in the allocation of resources to the NHS. If this structured change is to be implemented, savings in other areas of the health service would therefore have to be made. The alternatives appear to be (a) a reduction in the total number of doctors, thus creating doctor unemployment, or (b) a reduction in the medical school intake in order to reduce the bottleneck about to occur in the existing staffing structure. However, the effects of any change in present policy on medical school intake are subject to a time-lag of at least 6 years, owing to the training period.

It is clear that without an increase in real resource allocation to meet the increased cost of making the structural change, the demand for doctors, as constrained by future resource availability, will be exceeded by the supply of doctors. This would lead to doctor unemployment arising out of deficient demand. Clearly, such an outcome is significantly different from the frictional unemployment in the words of Engleman (see [26]), "a means to mobility within the profession", and hence not a bad thing and structural unemployment predicted by current conventional wisdom.

It is this fear of unemployment which has led the junior hospital doctors to demand a reduction in medical school intake, in addition to controls on doctor immigration. This contrasts with the Government's apparent abdication of responsibility for future manpower imbalances, as implied in a comment by the Chairman of the Short Committee (see [26]), who stated: " . . . no one knows how many doctors are needed by most certainly the Department (of Health and Social Security) do not intend to introduce a rigid notion of how many doctors should be trained. It is a matter for the profession as a whole including the medical schools and Royal Colleges."

No doubt the self-interest of the profession will lead to policy changes in the near future. Without such changes, doctor unemployment is likely to continue to grow from its present modest level of 2000 (in 1983).

References

1. Ministry of Health and Department of Health for Scotland (1944) Report of Interdepartmental Committee on Medical Schools, HMSO, London
2. Ministry of Health (1957) Report of the Committee to consider the future numbers of medical practitioners and the appropriate intake of medical students, HMSO, London
3. Abel-Smith B, Gales K (1964) British doctors at home and abroad. Codicote Press, Watford
4. Royal Commission on Medical Education (1968) Report (Chairman Lord Todd), HMSO, London (Cmnd. 3569)
5. Royal Commission on the National Health Service (1979) Report (Chairmann Sir Alec Merrison) HMSO, London (Cmnd. 7615)
6. Maynard A, Walker A (1978a) Doctor Manpower 1975–2000: alternative forecasts and their resource implications. Royal Commission on the National Health Service, Research Paper No. 4, HMSO, London
7. D.H.S.S. (1978) Medical manpower – the next twenty years. HMSO, London
8. D.H.S.S. (1980) Treasury and Central Policy Review Staff. Medical Manpower Steering Group Report (no publisher)
9. Maynard A, Walker A (1977) Too many doctors? Lloyds Bank Review 125, 24–36
10. Maynard A, Walker A (1978b) Medical manpower planning in Britain; a critical appraisal. In: Culyer AJ, Wright KG (eds) Economic Aspects of Health Services. Martin Robertson, London
11. D.H.S.S. (1976) Priorities for health and personal social services in England, HMSO, London

12. D.H.S.S. (1977) Priorities in the Health and Social Services. HMSO, London
13. O.P.C.S. (1980) Population projections, 1978–2018. HMSO, London
14. C.S.O. (1983) Economic Trends, HMSO, London
15. Reinhardt UE (1975) Physicians productivity and the demand for health manpower. Ballinger
16. Pauly MV (1980) Doctors and their workshops. National Bureau of Economic Research. University of Chicago Press, Chicago London
17. D.H.S.S. (1982) Health and Personal Social Service Statistics for England. HMSO, London
18. Scottish Home and Health Department (1981) Scottish Health Statistics. HMSO, London
19. Welsh Office (1983) Health and Personal Social Service Statistics for Wales, 1982, Welsh Office, Cardiff
20. D.H.S.S. (1983) Medical and dental staffing prospects in the N.H.S. in England and Wales, 1982, Health Trends, Vol. 15, 2, 35–39
21. Parkhouse J, Campbell MG, Parkhouse HF (1983) Career preferences of doctors qualifying in 1974–1980: a comparison of pre-registration findings. Health Trends, vol. 15, 2, 29–34
22. Ward A (1981) Careers of medical women. Medical Care Research Unit, University of Sheffield, Sheffield
23. Day P (1982b) Women Doctors: Choice and constraints in policies for medical manpower. Kings Fund Project Paper, London
24. Short R (1981) Fourth Report from the Social Services Committee 1980–1981. Medical Education with special reference to the number of doctors and the career structure in hospitals. HMSO, London
25. Clarke K (1982) The Government's response to the Select Committee's Report in P. Day (1982a)
26. Day P (1982a) Medical Manpower – the opportunity for change? King's Fund Report, London

Problems Related to Future Medical Demography in the European Community

A. Ritsatakis

1 Health Planning and Medical Manpower Planning

1.1 Definition of Health and Health Planning

The World Health Organization's often-quoted definition of health is "a stage of complete physical, mental and and social well-being and not merely the absence of disease or infirmity" (1). This broad definition is, however, a difficult one for planners to work with. In 1977, the 30th World Health Assembly agreed that an attempt should be made to attain for all citizens, by the year 2000, a level of health that would permit them to lead a socially and economically productive life (2). As a health planning objective, this is perhaps more concrete, but as is the nature of planning objectives, it still represents a broad concept, at a considerable distance from the actual setting of health planning targets.

The concept of planning for "health" as defined by "health for all by the year 2000" (HFA 2000) entails a multisectoral, multidisciplinary approach. In addition to health services, it must encompass questions of life-styles, such as smoking, eating and drinking habits, exercise or the lack of it; living standards, including income, housing and working conditions; physical and man-made environmental conditions; education etc.; demographic changes and particularly the aging of the population; and even questions such as personal and family relationships and levels of life-satisfaction.

In recent years, international bibliographies have been rich in references to planning for health rather than simply planning for health services, and international meetings, conferences and workshops touching on this matter have been equally abundant. So far, however, despite the acceptance of the WHO HFA 2000 proposals, there still seems to be an important gap between the exchange of ideas in the academic field and at international meetings, and the actual practice of health planning at the national level.

It should be evident that the provision of health services is not an end in itself, but one of the many means of achieving an improved level of health for the population. Since physicians are one of the main providers of health services, the demand for medical manpower is derived from the demand for such services. A WHO definition states that "Health manpower planning is the process of estimating the number of persons and the kind of knowledge, skills and attitudes they need to achieve predetermined health targets and ultimately health status objectives." (3)

However, the national papers in this study show, in the planning for medical manpower in many of the EEC countries, there still seems to be a danger of losing sight of the ultimate objective. Planning for health services appears more concrete and easy to deal with than planning for health. Questions of social demand for education, the need to employ existing stocks of medical manpower, entrenched methods of delivery health care, and the pressure and interest of the medical schools and the medical establishment appear to be the dominant forces. Consequently, out attention is perforce concentrated firstly on questions of planning for the health services.

1.2 Planning for Health Services

1.2.1 Peculiarities of the Health Services Sector

The health services differ from most other services in that many people believe that they should be provided according to need rather than to demand backed by willingness and ability to pay.

Rising expectations and improved education have made the population at large less willing to tolerate inferior standards and more reluctant to accept that particular sections of the community should be excluded from access to the medical care system. On the other hand, spiralling costs have made citizens, as taxpayers, ask whether cuts should be made somewhere.

In entering their profession, medical and nursing personnel are sworn to do their utmost protect and sustain life. Medical tradition emphasises to the provision of the best care that is technically possible, the only legitimate and explicitly recognised constraint being the state of the art, whereas suppliers of other services or products would be out of business if they did not weigh potential improvements against potential costs (4).

In recent years, with low rates of economic growth and increasing costs in the health sector, there seems to have been an almost overwhelming interest in reducing the resources used for health (5).

The financial resources allocated to the health sector depend on total resources available, economic growth and the competing demands of other sectors. The methods used to allocate resources to the health sector can vary from crude evaluations by policy-makers to highly sophisticated statistical models, particularly in countries where comprehensive development planning is carried out. Even the most sophisticated statistical methods, however, are fraught with value judgements, and in the final analysis, the amount of resources to be earmarked for health can only be the result of a political decision. The freedom exercised in such a decision is often narrowly restricted by the status quo, most decisions being of necessity incremental in nature.

The level of health spending in each country, however, seems to be determined more by its history than by more rational criteria. Furthermore, a higher level of health spending does not necessarily ensure a higher level of health, which, as mentioned above, is the final objective. Neither does it necessarily ensure a higher level of health services if it is simply absorbed in higher salaries for health personnel, for instance.

To take an example, the United Kingdom has a lower level of health spending than many developed countries, but conventionally used indicators show the level of health to be little different from that in those other countries. Life expectancy at birth in England, for example, although lower than in Sweden, the Netherlands and Denmark, is broadly the same as in France and Canada but higher than in the Federal Republic of Germany, Australia and the United States (6).

Similarly, the system of health care delivery does not seem to make much difference to the health status of the population in developed countries, as measured by conventional indicators (7). The demand for health services can, however, be affected by the health services system.

1.2.2 Need and Demand

Health status and the need for health services become more meaningful in terms of an individual's environment. For example, a person whose job requires him to read small print will probably become aware of a sight problem sooner than, say, an agricultural worker and will demand care to rectify the problem. Differentiation must be made between the need and the demand for health services, and between different types of need.

"Perceived illness" relates to the individual's subjective assessment of his own health status. There arises a "perceived need for care" when the individual translates his perception of his health status into demand for health care. "Professionally specified need" is the physician's assessment of the need for care, while "comparative need" relates to the morbidity of a group which has not come to the attention of the medical services, but whose existence is inferred by comparing it to another group whose needs are known (8).

The demand for health care will be determined, in most cases, firstly by the patient who presents himself for care, and then mainly by the physician through follow-up examination of the patient or referral to other health services.

Another aspect of the health services which make them different from many other services is that in many cases, demand seems to increase with supply. Roemer seems to have been one of the first to suggest that demand for hospital beds increases with supply, and this was borne out by Forsyth and Logan and others in later studies, all of whom came to the conclusion that the number of beds "used" or "demanded" is the number of beds available (9).

As mentioned above, apart from the patient who presents himself for care, medical personnel mainly determine the demand for health care. They do this by asking the patient to return so that his progress can be monitored, by ordering tests etc., by referring the patient to another physician, by authorizing hospital admittance, physiotherapy and rehabilitation services, etc. This cycle of referrals and demands for further health services occurs at different levels of the health services, depending on the first point of contact and the referral system of any particular health service system, but in any system, it is mainly the physician who is the key to demand. In other words, the medical personnel are largely responsible for modulating demand for their own and for other health services. Medical personnel in most countries have been very jealous in guarding their clinical autonomy, i.e. their right to determine how the patient can best be cared for, and the patient himself is in a weak position compared with the consumer in other sectors, since he does not have the necessary knowledge to evaluate what is best for him.

In planning for health services a pragmatic approach is frequently adopted, particularly where the public sector is not well developed. On the basis of the experience and intuitive skill of the decision-maker, rather than on clearly defined methodological concepts and techniques of analysis, step-by-step modifications are made to the health system. An inflexible legacy is frequently the main cause of this incremental approach. One of the main dangers of such an approach is that the lack or concrete data on which to base decisions makes them vulnerable to political pressures.

At the other end of the scale, various attempts have been, and are being, made to bring health planning into the realm of "scientific objectivity", such as the PAHO Cendes or Santiago methodology, which despite its weaknesses, is considered to be one of the most thorough attempts at applying systems analysis to the planning of health services (10).

1.2.3 Medical Manpower Planning

As in other fields of planning, there is a need in medical manpower planning to balance supply and demand. The social dissatisfaction caused by a shortage of medical manpower as manifested in long waiting lists, overcrowding or hasty consultations on the one hand, and the problems cause by large-scale unemployment of medical manpower on the other hand are evidence of the need for such a balance.

However, the achievement of a balance between supply and demand is not a simple matter either in the short or in the long term. In view of the length of time needed to train medical manpower, supply in the short term is largely determined by the existing stock of physicians and the number of students already in the education system. A specialist, for example, undergoes a total of about 12 years' medical training. Over the short term, therefore, it is difficult to change the level of supply, unless mass migration is envisaged. In other words, the possible supply of medical manpower is, to all intents and purposes, already determined for the year 2000.

Over both the short and the long term, supply is inevitably related to what can be a sensitive question of freedom of choice and the right to education.

When considering the long term, medical manpower planners must refer to more distant horizons than many other manpower planners. Over the periods of as long as 20 or 30 years which this may entail, many of the determinants of demand become increasingly difficult to estimate.

2 Summary of the National Papers

2.1 The Stock of Medical Manpower and Its Demographic Characteristics

There are at the present time about 504 500 active physicians in the ten countries of the EEC region. Spain and Portugal, which recently joined the EEC, have a further 127 000 physicians.

The number of inhabitants per physician varies from 775 in the United Kingdom to just over 600 in Luxenbourg, about 500 in the Netherlands, about 420 in Denmark, the Federal Republic of Germany, France and Ireland, 380 in Belgium and about 360 in Greece. The two new members of the Community – Spain and Portugal – have about 360 and 450 inhabitants per active physician, respectively.

It is clear from the above that the less economically developed EEC countries, which are also those with the shortest tradition of a large public sector, are the ones with the largest supply of active physicians in relation to the size of their population.

In the six countries which supplied information concerning the age of doctors (Denmark, Federal Republic of Germany, France, Greece, Italy and United Kingdom) young doctors under 40 years of age account for 40% and over of the total stock in most cases. In the United Kingdom, young doctors accounted for fully 65% of the total stock in 1981. The increasing proportion of young doctors in the total stock over the past 20 years is apparent in all six countries, Italy reporting an increase in very young doctors (34 years old or younger) from less than 25% in 1973 to more than 50% in 1984. Denmark, however, expects that over the next 20 years the proportion of young doctors will fall from its present 50% to about 25%.

Age can affect the services which medical manpower is able to offer, from the point of view of experience on the one hand and of ability to withstand arducus duties on the other. Concern is expressed with regard to the decrease in the proportion of the middle-age groups, which comprise the physicians upon whom the heaviest responsibilities are placed.

With regard to equality between the sexes, there is still a long way to go, and even by the end of the century women will not account for 50% of medical manpower. In this respect, although the relevant data are not entirely complete, Greece appears to be in the most favourable position with about 35% of physicians being women, compared to only about 16% in the United Kingdom, for example. It has been suggested that the comparatively high participation rate of women in the professions in some economically less developed countries has been partly due to the fact that women were able more easily to find substitute care for young children and continued to work when married (11), a situation which is now changing in those countries.

The position is improving, however, with an increasing proportion of women among very young doctors and among medical students. Denmark, for example, expects that women will account for 50% of medical graduates during the 1980s.

2.2 Education and Training of Medical Manpower

2.2.1 Undergraduate Education

In all the countries in the study, the undergraduate education of physicians is the responsibility of the Ministry of Education, and in most cases, the individual medical schools are responsible for the curriculum.

Undergraduate education lasts 5–6 years, including a period of training after graduation which is compulsory prior to registration as a physician. In the United Kingdom, for example, undergraduate education lasts 5 years and comprises two years of basic science and three years of clinical work. Graduation is followed by a year of study (six months' medicine and six months' surgery) prior to registration with the General Medical Council. In Denmark, this basic training includes an additional 6 months in general practice.

The countries taking part in the study, except Italy and Belgium, reported an attempt to limit the undergraduate intake.

A *numerus clausus* system has been in effect in France, for example, since 1972 and has been considerably tightened since 1978. Owing to the more open university system in France, however, restrictions are imposed by the state in the second years. In other words, all those qualified are entitled to enrol in the first year of medical school. At the end of that year, however, students undergo examination, and the government determines the number to be allowed to enrol in the second year.

Similarly, in Denmark, admission to medical school has been limited since 1976, and the intake has been progressively restricted in the 1980s. As in France, students are re-assessed after their first year. About 80% of them progress to the second year and most of these later graduate.

Both Greece and Ireland, however, report that although entrance to medical school is supposedly restricted, the targets set are in fact considerably exceeded. In Greece in particular, large numbers of students enter medical schools by the back-door, transferring from foreign universities in the second year, and preferential treatment is given to certain special groups such as children of war victims, refugees, etc., who further swell the number of students admitted.

In Italy, the number of medical students is greatly expanded by the intake of foreign students. It is estimated that in 1977, for example, there were about 10 000 foreign medical students studying in Italy.

The problems of overcrowding in medical schools and the detrimental effects on the quality of education were emphysised in the national papers. It is suggested that even when the intake of new medical students is restricted, this is not always related to the training capacity of the university or to the demands of modern medical education. Rather harsh criticism from the Federal Republic of Germany suggests that the intake is not related to training capacity in that country and even less to the demand for physicians.

Finally, there appears to be some concern about the content of the undergraduate curriculum. In some cases, there is a fear that changes are too often simply additive and that in the southern European countries where technical equipment and facilities in relation to the number of students are comparatively poor, this has led to an over-emphasis on theoretical education.

2.2.2 Postgraduate Education and Specialist Training

Whereas in the case of undergraduate education the role of the Ministry of Education is dominant, in the case of postgraduate or specialist training there is a shift of responsibility, with the Ministry of Health or its equivalent, and also in some cases the medical associations, moving to the fore. In the Federal Republic of Germany, the federal government is responsible for the laws on the education of physicians, but the states are responsible for monitoring the practice of medicine. This means that the states have responsibility for continuing and postgraduate education in both general and special medicine. In the United Kingdom, responsibility for arranging in-training examinations lies with the Royal Colleges.

The shift in responsibility with regard to undergraduate and postgraduate education is felt to cause a lack of continuity in medical education, and there is perhaps some lack of relevance between the two stages.

Postgraduate education for general practice is not available in all cases (in Italy, for example, there is no postgraduate training for general practitioners, whereas in Ireland there is a programme but it is not compulsory for general practice), but where it is, such education takes about a further 3 years. For hospital specialists on the other hand, there is an additional training period of 5–6 years and even 5–8 years. It is estimated in Denmark, for example, that whereas university training ends typically around the age of 27–28, specialists are usually in their late 30s before they complete their training. The amount of effort and human and economic resources sunk into the training of such specialists is self-evident.

Entrance to postgraduate training is regulated by limiting the number of training positions available. In Italy, for example, it is estimated that the positions available each year represent less than 20% of the annual number of qualified medical students.

The very high competition for these limited positions is considered in Denmark to have contributed to an improvement in the quality of specialists being trained, since only the best graduates are able to progress to such training. On the other hand, there is perhaps a danger in the creation of large pools of dissatisfied physicians, particularly if this means that the best are creamed off for the hospitals, leaving the "unsuccessful" ones to fill positions in the primary care services.

There appears to be no marked evidence of planning for the training of specialists on the basis of demand and supply. On the whole, it appears that the limiting of positions for specialist training is linked more to considerations of the facilities available for training in existing hospitals than to the expected demand for particular specialities. Some countries, as for example France and more recently Greece, have been curtailing the number of positions for specialist training in an attempt to divert more young physicians towards general practice.

2.3 Present Employment of Medical Manpower

The uneven regional distribution of medical manpower appears to be a problem in all the countries of the EEC, physicians being mainly concentrated in urban areas. In Denmark, for example, whereas there are only 200 inhabitants per physician in the capital, the figure is 600–700 in western Denmark, and in 1982 some areas had a 25% deficiency in their quota of physicians. Similarly, in Italy, the highest density of doctors is in Rome. There are 148 inhabitants per physician in provincial capital towns and 403 inhabitants per physician in the remainder of the country. In Greece, this maldistribution is particularly pronounced, with 57% of physicians concentrated in the Great Athens area and a ratio of inhabitants to physician ranging from 226 in the capital to 1330 in Central Greece and Euboea. In the United Kingdom, on the other hand, it is some of the large urban areas, where industrialization had deteriorated the living environment, which are in an inferior position, compared to some less urbanised areas which many physicians consider to be desirable residential areas.

Most of the EEC countries appear to have been grappling unsuccessfully with this problem for many years, implementing systems of incentives to attract physicians to areas with insufficient medical manpower. In the United Kingdom, in addition to such incentives, restrictions are placed on the registration of new physicians in areas which are considered to be over-supplied. In Greece, under a law passed over twenty years ago and still in effect, graduates of the medical schools must undergo a period of compulsory service in rural surgeries. Although this has had the effect of keeping the rural surgeries open, it has meant that the rural population are frequently provided with a comparatively low level of primary care by inexperienced young physicians.

This uneven distribution relates to physicians in both primary and hospital care. In the United Kingdom in 1980, for example, the number of hospital physicians per 100 000 inhabitants ranged from 69.9 to 98.6 and that of general practitioners from 47.6 to 57.1

A certain amount of variation in the employment of physicians in different areas is natural, owing to the concentration of specialized hospital services in certain urban areas, which, however, serve a much wider population than that in the immediate vicinity, and to the employment in urban areas of physicians in non-clinical positions, i.e. in administrative, teaching or research positions. It is not the existence of uneven distribution which is at fault, but the degree of inequality when this means that some population groups are receiving health services vastly inferior to those received by others.

Throughout the EEC countries, the number of hospital doctors has been increasing faster than that of those in general practice. In the Federal Republic of Germany, for example, there were 23 000 physicians in hospitals in 1960 and nearly 67 500 by 1981. Similarly, in Italy, whereas there were 16.5 hospital beds per physician in 1961, by 1981 there were only 6.4 beds per physician.

The proportion of physicians employed in hospitals obviously varies with the system of health care delivery. Fully 60% of physicians are employed in hospitals in Denmark, 25% are general practitioners and 15% are in school medical services, social services, administration or the universities. In Greece, 51% of physicians were employed in hospitals and clinics in 1982, although many were simultaneously employed in primary care, whereas in the Federal Republic of Germany, 41.2% are employed full-time in hospitals.

As will be seen from the following section, the terms of employment for physicians vary enormously, from salaried positions for most hospital doctors and for some doctors in primary care to systems such as fee-for-service, fee-per-visit, fee-per-hour, per capita remuneration or various mixes of these.

The distribution of physicians between the public and the private sector also varies considerably, as might be expected, but even in countries with a national health service, the proportion of physicians in private practice can be considerable. In France, 68% of physicians are in private practice, and in the Federal Republic of Germany this proportion is 35%, with the number in private practice increasing. In Italy and the United Kingdom, a number of physicians employed in the national health services of those countries are also engaged in private practice. Under 60% of physicians in public hospitals in Italy are employed full-time, 40% working a 28-hour week and working also in private practice or in out-patient departments; in addition, there are a number of doctors in private hospitals contracted to the national health service (16% of total beds in Italy are private, contracted to the national health service). Only in Greece is it considered that private practice should be totally prohibited for those employed in the national health service.

2.4 Trends in the Balance of Supply and Demand

Without exception, all the countries taking part in the study report a very rapid increase in the supply of doctors in recent years. The number of active physicians in Denmark more than doubled betwen 1960 and 1980. France also reports very rapid growth, with the result that the number of physicians per 100 000 inhabitants more than doubled between 1965 and 1983, increasing from 112 to 236. Similarly, in the Federal Republic of Germany, the increase in the number of graduates continues to exceed the increase in the population. In Greece, at the time of the formulation of the 1976–1980 Development Plan, it was already considered that the excess supply of physicians was detrimental to the quality of the health services, because of the undesirable competition which it created. The supply of physicians in Italy quadrupled between 1954 and 1984, with the number of doctors per 1000 population increasing from 1.2 to 3.8. Finally, in the United Kingdom in the 7-year period 1974–1981 alone, the number of hospital physicians increased by 24.5% and that of general practitioners by 13.1%.

In many of the EEC countries, there appears to have been a shortage of physicians in the 1960s as the health services and public insurance schemes were expanded during a period of rapid economic growth. With the onset of the economic crisis during the 1970s and a tightening of the resources earmarked for health, this shortage was transformed into a surplus.

In France, the Sixth Social and Economic Development Plan (1971–1975), for example, estimated that 200 active physicians per 100 000 population would be needed by 1985, but this level had already been reached by 1979. A study ordered by the Federal Ministry of Labour and Social Affairs in 1979 estimated that as far as could reasonably be calculated, an additional 20 000–25 000 professionally active physicians would be required in the Federal Republic of Germany between 1978 and the year 2000, and that demand would therefore fall far short of the expected increase in the supply of physicians.

Consequently, unemployment or underemployment of physicians is already in evidence. It is estimated in Italy, for example, that 20% of the total registered physicians under 70 years of age are unemployed or underemployed, i.e. almost 1.0 physician per 1000 population.

2.5 Migration

In some cases, part of the problem of balancing supply and demand appears to have been met by the migration of physicians. The United Kingdom seems to represent a particular case in which considerable numbers of British doctors emigrated to the United States, mainly in search of higher remuneration, and physicians from less developed countries, particularly those of the Commonwealth, flowed into the British health service to fill the gap, a manifestation of what has been called the "brain drain". Restrictions on health expenditure in the United States, however, have greatly reduced the flow across the Atlantic. Similarly, there has been a reduction in the proportion of doctors born overseas practising in the United Kingdom, from 35% in 1974 to 31.4% in 1981. For years, the overflow of physicians from Ireland was also absorbed by the United States, Canada and Australia, but this has now become much more difficult. It was estimated in 1982 that 12% of the total number of authorized Danish doctors were resident outside Denmark, mainly in Norway and Sweden. Medical migration flows into and out of France, on the other hand, are not very significant, and this situation is expected to contiue during the 1980s.

Under EEC directives first proposed in 1969, adopted in 1975 and operational since 1976, doctors in the EEC – whether specialists or general practitioners, self-employed or salaried – can practise in all member countries. The basic training of qualified doctors must include at least 6 years of higher education or 5500 hours of theoretical or practical study. The contents of the training course are not laid down. Specialists must have followed an additional training course of 3–5 years (12).

The migration of physicians within the EEC can be seen from Table 1. For each year, the first column shows physicians who are nationals of the country from which they received authorization to practise, i.e. they are physicians who received their basic medical education abroad (in an EEC country) and returned home to practise. The second column shows physicians who are nationals of a member state other than the one in which they received their authorization. As can be seen, the total movement of doctors within the

Table 1. Number of doctors who are nationals of an EEC member country and who obtained their basic qualification in another member country, whose authorization to practise was issued 1977–1983 (from [13])

Country awarding authorization	1977 (a)	1977 (b)	1978 (a)	1978 (b)	1979 (a)	1979 (b)	1980 (a)	1980 (b)	1981 (a)	1981 (b)	1982 (a)	1982 (b)	1983 (a)	1983 (b)
Federal Republic of Germany	3	242	3	269	11	370	7	350	23	455[e]	24	491[f]	7	1011
France	24	47	6	42	5	34	5	40	12	40	15	81	12	58
Italy[c]	. .	. .	1	–	6	27	7	19	–	17	1	24	2	20
Netherlands	–	121	10	79	13	63	1	33	31	62	29	47	17	28
Belgium	5	14	6	16	2	18	2	24	2	12	–	13	4	15
Luxembourg[d]	. .	14	. .	8	. .	13	. .	12	. .	12	. .	8	. .	7
United Kingdom	14	437	8	462	6	409	5	395	7	539	7	622	10	557
Ireland	–	40	–	47	–	31	–	81	–	57	1	37	–	35
Denmark	–	11	–	12	1	6	1	5	–	6	–	6	–	9
Greece	. .	. .	. .	. .	. .	. .	. .	. .	111	18	230	16	390	12
Total	46	926	34	935	44	971	28	959	186	1218	307	1345	442	1752

Those who have acquired authorization to practise in the country of their basic medical education are excluded, since they are affectively migrant students. Those who have authorization and are continuing with specialized studies are included, except for France and Luxembourg, where migrants can specialize without having received authorization.

(a) Nationals of country in which authorization was received. (b) Nationals of country other than that in which authorization was received.
[c] Law transforming Directives on doctors into national legislation not adopted until May 1978.
[d] Since all Luxenbourg students have to train in other countries, the table does not include students who return.
[e] Except Hesse.
[f] Unlike the other countries, this figure includes doctors of other member countries who, having obtained their qualifications in the Federal Republic of Germany, have established themselves there.
. . not applicable.

EEC in any one year is not very large, nor is it expected to be, particularly in view of the language barriers between some of the countries.

The analytical tables (13) from which these data are taken show this movement of doctors by their country of origin and by the country in which they received their basic medical education. From those tables, it can be seen that the majority of physicians from member countries, authorized to practise in the United Kingdom, were from Ireland. The Irish accounted for over 80% of such physicians in 1977, and although this proportion had fallen to just over 40% in 1983, the numbers of Irish doctors moving to the United Kingdom remained around the 250–350 level, the proportional drop being partly due to the inclusion of Greece in the tables after 1981. Greek nationals accounted for 24% of EEC physicians receiving their authorization in the United Kingdom in 1983. Almost all physicians from EEC countries, authorized to practise in Ireland, during this period were from the United Kingdom. No other equally strong bilateral flows are evident. Belgian physicians predominate in the flow towards the Netherlands, and Greece accounts for 35%–40% of EEC physicians who have received authorization in the Federal Republic of Germany since 1981. With regard to Greece itself, over 95% of those authorized after studying and qualifying in another country are Greek nationals returning home, mainly from Italy, the Federal Republic of Germany and the United Kingdom.

2.6 Medical Manpower Planning in the EEC Countries

In most cases, it is explicitly stated in the national papers that medical manpower planning has been related more to training capacity and economic resources that to the supply of and demand for health services.

As alread stated, the health services are a rather peculiar case in which demand seems to increase with supply. In Denmark, the number of consultations has increased parallel to the number of doctors, and the Danish paper states that it is not apparent to what extent growth in the number of physicians corresponds to need.

The recent restrictions on the intake of medical students in Frace have been based mainly on economic grounds, not on grounds of "unnecessary" provision of health services. Indeed, although such negative aspects as the undue power of the physician and the over-consumption of drugs have been widely debated, it is stated that there is a consensus of both left- and right-wing political parties that most demand is justified. At the same time, it is pointed out in the French paper that it is generally accepted that the supply of medical manpower is not related to the level of health.

The paper from the Federal Republic of Germany, quoting a special study carried out in that country, suggests that an "objective, unequivocal (estimation of the) demand for physicians does not exist".

Where attempts have been made to relate planning for the education of physicians to the needs of the health services for medical manpower, this appears to have been done mainly by projecting past trends of utilization of services, with adjustments for demographic changes, into the framework of existing patterns of services. The weaknesses of such methods, as well as failure to relate medical manpower planning to possible changes in the structure and organisation of health services, have been pointed out very forcefully in the British national paper. In a similar vein, the Greek paper suggests that a change in the responsibilities and duties carried out by physicians in Greece could greatly affect the need for medical manpower.

3 National Frameworks

3.1 Population and Health Statistics

The question of medical manpower cannot be looked at in a vacuum, but must be seen in a national and a Community framework.

The EEC, including Spain and Portugal, which jointed the Community in January 1986, now has a population of about 320 million. Table 2 shows the heterogeneity in the size of the member countries, their populations ranging from 366 000 in Luxembourg to 61 million in the Federal Republic of Germany.

However, as indicated in a recent study by the Organization for Economic Co-operation and Development (14) from which the data for Table 2 are taken, there are no very large discrepancies in life expectancy in the member countries. It is interesting to note that comparatively favourable position of the southern European countries in this respect.

The infant mortality rate, however, which is said to be more closely related to the level of health services than is life expectancy, does show wide variations, the level of 7.7 infant deaths per 1000 life births in Denmark being less than half that in Greece and Portugal, for example.

The proportion of elderly people in the Community is increasing, particularly that of the very old, who tend to make heavy use of the health services. Much of the gain in life expectancy at age 60 occurred before 1950. Although there has been little or no change for elderly males in more recent years, among females there are continous steady increments in life expectancy at age 60 in almost all countries (15).

The increasing proportion of the elderly, and particularly the very old, affects not only the amount of health services which will be required but also the type of services and whether these can be provided in the home or in an institutional setting. In Europe in 1980, for every 100 persons aged 60–64, there were an estimated 55 persons aged 80 and over (16). Multigenerational families are becoming numerous, many of them having elderly members of two generations, with surviving octogenarians who live with children in their 60s. In other word, in many cases the old are caring for the very old, and it is in such a family setting that health care must be provided.

Furthermore, health care must be provided in a setting in which the traditional home care-givers, i.e. the female population, are achieving higher participation rates in employment, even when they have young children.

3.2 Health Care Delivery

3.2.1 Belgium

The Kingdom of Belgium has four linguistic regions, is divided into three communities – Flemish, French and German – and has three political regions. According to the con-

Table 2. Population (1983), life expectancy (1980) and infant mortality (1983) in EEC countries (from [14])

Member state	Population (thousands)	Life expectancy 1980 At birth		At age 40		At age 60		Infant deaths per 1000 live births
	1983	Males	Females	Males	Females	Males	Femals	1983
Federal Republic of Germany	61 421	69.7	76.5	32.9	38.6	16.4	20.7	10.3
France	54 438	70.1	78.3	33.2	40.2	17.2	22.3	8.9
Italy	56 835	70.7	77.4	33.7	39.5	17.1	21.3	12.4
Netherlands	14 362	72.5	79.2	34.7	40.7	17.5	22.7	8.4
Belgium	9 856	69.8	75.5	32.0	37.5	15.5	20.0	11.2
Luxembourg	366	68.0	75.1	31.3	37.1	15.1	19.8	11.2
United Kingdom	56 377	70.2	75.9	32.7	38.2	15.9	20.5	10.2
Ireland	3 508	69.5	75.0	32.0	36.2	15.5	18.8	9.8
Denmark	5 114	71.4	77.6	33.9	39.2	17.2	21.7	7.7
Greece	9 850	73.2	77.8	36.4	40.1	19.0	21.7	14.6
Spain	38 228	71.5	78.0	34.5	39.6	18.0	21.0	9.6[a]
Portugal	10 058	67.0	75.0	32.0	38.0	16.0	20.0	19.0

[a] 1982 figure.

stitution, the communities are responsible for matter "concerning the public". and this includes health policy. However, the national government fixes the norms and each community governments applies them (17).

The lack of clear division of authority between the national administration and the communities has created a number of problems. Further problems of co-ordination are caused by the fact that a global health policy has not yet been defined, measures being carried out in individual sectors through legislation and regulation under separate laws and through separate advisory bodies for each sector and area of concern (i.e. mother and child care, tuberculosis prevention, industrial medical services, etc.). This piecemeal approach means that various pressure groups are able to exert an inordinate amount of influence on policy.

Most of the health establishments in Belgium (hospitals, psychiatric institutions, health centres, services for mental health care, nursing homes for the elderly, etc.) are non-profit religious organizations or private institutions, the latter being only a small minority. They have the legal status of other non-profit organizations, operate in general without any form of co-operation and are not co-ordinated with the public sector, which provides care for certain groups through the Public Centres for Community Welfare and through municipal hospitals.

Primary care is provided by independent private practitioners. General practitioners and, to a large extent, specialists provide care in their own surgeries, group practices not having been developed very much so far. Specialists also provide care in separate or hospital-based out-patient departments, and patients have direct access to their services.

The preventive and curative health services are separated administratively, physically and financially, and with regard to their staffing.

There is a compulsory sickness and disability insurance scheme which is the responsibility of the state, but is run by private non-profit sickness funds and covers most of the costs of health care. It has been suggested that in recent years "health insurance has made as it were a 'coup d'etat' on health policy. Health insurance does not restrict itself any more to the financing of health care but determines to quite an extent which care may or can be provided to the public and under which conditions and in what circumstances" (18). This use of the social security system indirectly to guide the development of the health care system by granting or withholding reimbursement for given types of care has taken place without an overall strategy (19).

3.2.2 Denmark

The Ministry of the Interior is responsible for health in Denmark (20). Working in close collaboration with this ministry is the National Board of Health, which is a civil service unit. The National Board of Health is, however, obliged to advise all ministries on health issues. It supervises the output of the health care system, being represented at the county level by public medical officers. There is also a committee under this Board to advise on the content of postgraduate specialist training.

There are two political/administrative levels under the national level – the counties and the municipalities – and taxes are raised at all levels. There is a very strong philosophy of deconcentration and decentralisation, with responsibility of public services being more and more delegated from state to county and municipal levels. Parliament has no legal right to interfere in the autonomy of the counties in their planning and running of health matters.

The state is responsible for legislation and therefore for the health care system and its supervision, the counties for planning and running most health care services and the municipalities for planning and running certain local and public health services.

Hospitals, general as well as psychiatric, are owned and run by the counties, and a special committee is responsible for co-ordinating hospital activities across county borders. There are very few private hospitals, and from the patient's point of view these are run as an integrated part of public hospital services in collaboration with the counties. Hospital treatment is free of charge to the patient, who is admitted only after referral from a physician or through the hospital emergency unit.

The public health insurance system is financed by taxes rather than contributions. A number of primary health care services are guaranteed either free or partly free, and the health insurance system partly reimburses the cost of a number of pharmaceutical products.

Medical personnel working under the public health insurance system retain a semi-independent position. They are responsible for establishing and running the service, and are paid a combination of fee-for-service and salary per capita. The general practitioner is the key person and the "gate-keeper" of the Danish system.

Ninety-five per cent of the population belong to the no-cost system, under which they have the right to change their doctor only once a year, less than 5% being in the co-payment scheme (Group II), under which there is an unrestricted choice of physician.

Home nursing, paediatric nursing, children's dentistry and school health care are provided by the municipalities.

3.2.3 France

The administrative and political dvisions in France are at the level of the region, department, administrative district (*arrondissement*) and the commune (21). The region is now a territorial authority managed by a Regional Council which is directly elected. The department is run jointly by an executive body, the Prefect and a directly elected General Council, and it is to this level that most services have been decentralised. The commune is a decentralised body, also run by a directly elected municipal council. Since 1982, there has been a move towards greater decentralisation.

The Ministry of Social Affairs and National Solidarity supervises the health services through its representatives at the regional level.

There is a very strong tradition of private non-profit organizations in France, and they continue to play an important role in the delivery of health services, together with the public sector, in primary, secondary and tertiary health care.

The Social Security Funds also have private law status and are financed by contributions. One of the main characteristics of this system is respect for the principles of free medicine. The social insurance institutions remain neutral regarding the relation of the patient to the doctor, confining themselves to the reimbursement of services freely chosen, subject to certain limits. In some cases, the insurance funds set up and directly manage certain health services, or finance the equipment and functioning of such services.

3.2.4 Federal Republic of Germany

In the Federal Republic of Germany (22), statutory sickness insurance covers health care for about 90% of the population. Federal law regulates the general framework of this system, including membership of the approximately 1300 sickness funds, access to services, financing and organization of the funds, organization of the physicians and dentists working for the funds, as well as their highly complicated mutual relationships.

The different sickness funds operate on a nationwide or local basis and may relate to regional boundaries or a single factory, to single branches of the economy or to employment status, i.e. blue- or white-collar workers. The various insurance fund organizations negotiate autonomously with the physician's and dentists' association concerning details of service delivery and remuneration, including monitoring of quality and cost-efficiency. There is little room left for public administration and governmental interference. Planning and financing in the hospital sector constitute the strongest field of state regulation and public administration.

Autonomy is a deeply rooted, fundamental principle in the Federal Republic of Germany's health system, which is not questioned by any of the political parties.

At the federal level, the Federal Ministry of Labour and Social Affairs and the Federal Ministry of Youth, Family Affairs and Health share responsibility for health policies. In the state governments, health is organizationally combined with various other policy fields.

There is a standing committe of state ministries with responsibility for health. The local governments and local government associations implement federal and state laws, and are the owner-operators of various health care facilities.

3.2.5 Greece

In Greece until recently there were only first-level local authorities, i.e. municipalities and communities, administered by council elected by direct vote (23). In July 1986 Law 1622 was passed, providing for the setting up of second- and third-level authorities at county and regional levels, and this law is to be implemented in the immediate future. Although the legal framework existing prior to 1986 gave the first-level local authorities considerable power to provide health services, owing to their very small size and lack of economic resources, few did in fact provide such services.

Most decision-making continues to be carried out at the central level or through government-appointed representatives (*nomarches*) at the level of the basic administrative unit, the *nomos* or county, which will now operate as the second-level local authority, with the *nomarchis* retaining much of his decisive authority.

In 1983, a law setting up a National Health System (NHS) was passed. Until the full implementation of this law, the system continues to operate as before, i.e. the rural population and urban workers are covered for primary and hospital care by their separate insurance organizations; together, they account for almost 70% of the population. A large number of insurance funds cover various other employment groups for health care, about 98% of the total population having some form of health insurance coverage.

The private health sector in Greece is still very strong, about 40% of total hospital beds being in private clinics. Under the law on the NHS, the establishment of new private clinics has been prohibited.

The delivery of primary health care varies according to the health insurance organization. Urban workers and the rural population receive care from family doctors or in the health centres run by their separate insurance funds, these physicians being employed on a salaried basis. Most of the other organizations use physicians contracted to them, who are renumerated on a fee-for-service or fee-for-consultation basis, either by the insurance fund or by the patient, who is then reimbursed.

For the most part, patients have direct access to specialists, with the result that the bulk of the work being done by many specialists in primary care would in most other European countries have been carried out by a general practitioner.

The Central Health Council, which was set up in 1982 and is composed of representatives of the medical associations, insurance funds, medical schools, local authorities, trade unions and the Ministry of Health, Welfare and Social Security, has the main responsibility for the definition of the general aims of health policy. It is also responsible for assessment of the professional activities of medical manpower. The boundaries of the Health Regions proposed for the NHS were defined in February 1986 and Regional Health Councils are to be set up at that level.

The state hospital services are to be regionalised, and health centres are being set up as outposts of those hospitals. The new system can be characterised as deconcentrated rather then decentralised. The health centres and hospital out-patient departments under the new system will accept patients referred to them by family doctors, or by appointment.

3.2.6 Italy

A National Health Service (NHS) was set up in Italy in 1978 (24). This system is decentralised, responsibility being distributed among the central, regional and local levels. The central level is responsible for health policy guidelines and for planning, financing and monitoring at the national level. The regions are responsible for planning primary and hospital care in their areas according to government health policy, and the communes and local health units must organize and run the services.

The Minister of Health has a number of health councils, institutes and committees at his disposal to assist in the formulation of health policy, and a national health plan is prepared every 3 years.

The regions have a considerable amount of autonomy in translating government health policy into technical and operational decisions. The Regional Health Departments vary in organization in different regions, some including social services and environmental or ecological planning in their field of responsibility.

The Local Health Unites (LHUs) constitute the operational level of the NHS and are directly dependent on one or more communes; some large cities have more than one LHU, Rome having 20, for example. The LHUs are managed by locally elected or appointed councils. For the purposes of primary care and co-ordination with social services, they are divided into districts, within which direct citizens' participation in health service management is to take place. These districts are not yet fully operational.

The public and private sectors work together within the framework of the NHS. General practitioners operate under an agreement with the NHS in their own private practices, being remunerated on a per capita basis. Agreement is reached at the national level between the government and the medical unions concerning tasks, responsibilities and fees, and the number of patients to be registered with each general practitioner. General practitioners may also accept non-registered patients on a private basis.

Specialists may operate in their own practices or in clinics owned by the LHUs, and are paid on a fee-for-service basis. Clinical analyses requested by a physician and authorised by the LHU can also be provided by private operators, who are paid through the NHS.

In areas where there are not enough public beds, the regions and local health districts may make agreements with private hospitals. The procedures for hospitalisation in these units are similar to those relating to public hospitals.

3.2.7 Ireland

Responsibility for health policy in Ireland lies with the Department of Health, whose Secretary is responsible to the *Dáil* (parliament) for ensuring that all monies voted for the health services are properly utilised for the purposes approved by law. There are no formal arrangements for co-ordinating the work of the Department of Health with other departments (25).

Non-governmental organizations feature prominently in the provision of hospital and institutional services, community-based health and welfare services, and a range of advisory, counselling and health education services. The voluntary hospitals and institutions provide services under an agreement with the health boards. For administrative convenience and owing to the long-standing relationship with these hospitals, discussions on budgetary targets and limits take place within the Department, and funding is channelled directly from the Department to the hospitals.

The main burden of operating the services is laid on the health boards, which are corporate bodies. These boards may act jointly in providing some services, co-operative with local authorities and enter into agreements with other bodies, such as the voluntary hospitals, to provide services on their behalf. About 52% of the members of these boards are public representatives, i.e. members of county councils in the boards' functional areas; the rest are elected representatives of the main health professions, and a small number of members are appointed by the Minister.

Each board, within the overall allocation made to it on an annual basis by the Department, would be free to redeploy resources between programmes and to determine its priorities for both capital and revenue developments. The boards cannot, however, embark on major capital developments, increase or upgrade their staffing, without prior approval of the Department, or replace or create medical consultant posts without the approval of the National Hospitals Council.

A person's eligibility for services depends on his financial status. Persons in Category I, who in the opinion of the chief executive officer of the health board are unable to afford general practitioner services, are entitled to the full range of health services without charge. Just under 40% of the population are in this category. About 45% are in Category II according to their income, and are entitled to hospital services in public wards, specialist services in out-patient clinics, and to infant welfare and maternity services. They are also entitled to a refund of part of the cost of prescribed medicines. The rest – in Category III – are entitled without charge to hospital services on the same basis as those in Category II, but are liable to pay hospital consultants' fees.

3.2.8 United Kingdom

A National Health Service (NHS) has been operating in the United Kingdom for 40 years (26). One of the main differences between this and similar services in other countries, in terms of public administration, is the apparent absence of clearly defined measures for the control and direction of health services by government and parliament. Essentially, the Department of Health and Social Security must rely on persuasion and exhortation in dealing with all the other central government departments with an indirect interest in health services.

The planning, management and delivery of services depend on an agency relationship between the responsible minister and the Department of Health and Social Security on the one hand, and the NHS operating sub-nationally through 14 Regional Health Authorities (RHAs) and 192 District Health Authorities (DHAs) on the other hand.

The NHS receives about 88% of its funds from general taxation, about 9% from insurance contributions and the rest mainly from charges to patients.

The latest reorganization of the NHS is intended to make local management stronger and more efficient. RHAs and DHAs are the main employers of NHS staff and to a large extent are free to decide their own mix of manpower and other resources, within the overall constraints of their cash limits.

The family doctor service and general dental, pharmaceutical and ophthalmic services are provided by independent practitioners contracted to 90 Family Practitioner Committees. The chairmen and members of these Committees are appointed by the DHAs, the local authorities and local professional committees.

The general practitioner is the first point of contact for the patient, who does not normally have direct access to the consultant. Increasingly, the GP now forms part of a multiprofessional primary health care team; whereas in 1969, 27% of unrestricted principals operated in partnerships of three or more, by 1981 this proportion had increased to 45%, and only 13% were operating single-handed.

Hospital and specialist services are managed by the DHAs, which are accountable to the RHAs. The main postgraduate teaching hospitals are each managed by a special Health Authority accountable directly to the Secretary of State for Health.

The local authorities have general responsibility for public health and a wide range of community-based services.

Despite the long life of the NHS, there has always been an independent health sector in the United Kingdom, and doctors have been allowed private practice in the NHS since its inception. Apart from the private hospitals, nursing homes and day clinics, nearly 700 public hospitals have a number of "pay beds" and nearly 850 NHS hospitals accept private out-patients.

Community Health Councils were established in 1974 to provide a means of representing public opinion. Their members are appointed by local authorities, voluntary organizations and the RHAs.

3.2.9 Luxembourg

Because of its limited territory, Luxembourg is centralised with regard to the administrative organization of health care, with the Minister of Health responsible for its administration throughout the country (27). He is advised by a Hospital Council established in 1977. The members of the Council are representatives of the government, the Medical College, the union of sickness benefit societies, the hospitals and the medical and paramedical professions.

Most of the population are insured with a health fund. All physicians established in the Grand Duchy automatically work within the framework of the social security system and are paid according to standard rates fixed by the health funds. Patients are reimbursed for 80% of general practitioners' fees, apart from antenatal and postnatal care, which are fully covered, and for 80% of the cost of most drugs.

Hospital care is provided in both public and private hospitals. With regard to the cost of hospitalization, insured persons contribute a fixed amount per day, except in the case of long-term care (mental illness, tuberculosis, cancer and poliomyelitis), which is covered by the state through the "heavy risk" insurance funds.

The Red Cross also plays a significant part in the provision of health care in Luxembourg.

3.2.10 Netherlands

In the Netherlands, the Ministry of Health, Welfare and Cultural Affairs is responsible for health, the minister being advised by a National Health Council (28). The Netherlands is divided into provinces, each administered by an elected Provincial Council. The municipality is the only form of administrative unit at the local service. For the purpose of the regionalization of the health services, the country is devided into 24 health regions.

Traditionally, health services in the Netherlands have been mainly in private hands, the government limiting its policy to the creation of conditions enabling private sector to organize the services and provide the care. Hospitals and other health service institutions are, therefore, mainly in private hands, although there are municipal institutions and state-run university hospitals. Private institutions have to comply with state regulations if they are to be financed from social security funds, and the quality of care has always been subject to state control.

Since the incorporation of the "right" to health care into the constitution in 1983, and with the rising cost of health care, there has been a move to reform health care on the basis of legislation, in the direction of deliberately chosen goals. Under the 1982 Health Services Act, provision was made for the Ministry of Health to prepare instructions for health policy to be implemented by the provinces and municipalities through their own health plans. The construction and running of health institutions is to be dependent on their inclusion in the approved provincial plans and on ministerial approval. The provincial governments are advised by Provincial Councils for Health, on which are represented health care institutions and workers, sickness funds, insurance companies, consumers, social welfare institutions and municipalities.

Under the 1981 Health Charges Act, it is not possible to charge different fees for the same services, although there may be differences under and outside an insurance scheme.

Agreements on hospital fees are concluded by the peripheral health insurance funds and the health services concerned, and are approved by the Central Health Charges Board. Fees for medical personnel outside hospitals and for specialists are decided by the representative organizations at the national level.

Various kinds of insurance schemes make health care facilities financially accessible – compulsory sick fund insurance, voluntary insurance, old people's insurance, supplementary insurance, private insurance, the state scheme for civil servants and compulsory insurance for special risks. The main compulsory scheme covers about 70% of the population for general health care, whereas the scheme for exceptional medical expenses in principle covers the whole population in respect of long-term care, nursing homes, services for the mentally handicapped, etc.

3.2.11 Summary and Conclusions

It can be seen from the above that in the EEC region, the United Kingdom has had a National Health Service for the longest period of time, and one which is lower on administrative costs than some other systems. The NHS does not appear, however, to have served as a means of ensuring the central government's direct control over the system. Italy has introduced a system which, although similar in some ways to that of the United Kingdom, is more decentralised. Greece is also in the process of setting up a NHS, but in a situation where the private sector is still very considerable.

The Federal Republic of Germany and Belgium, owing to the political and/or administrative structure of those countries, the system of health care delivery, is very decentralized, and indeed has been described as fragmented. The system in Denmark is also decentralized, the county councils having the main responsibility for directing both the hospital services and the insurance scheme.

In the Netherlands, the long tradition of mainly privately controlled health care is changing slightly, with the state taking a more important role. In all the EEC countries, there is a mixed system of public and private service, many of the private services, however, being covered by public insurance. Only in Greece has private practice for physicians employed in the public sector been completely prohibited.

The remuneration of physicians and their conditions of employment are as varied as the system. Hospital doctors in all systems are salaried, although some may also have other remuneration. Physicians working in primary care may be paid on a salaried, fee-for-service or per capita basis, or even on an hourly basis (as is the case for some specialists in Italy). There are also various mixes of these systems. Although some physicians in primary care are employed directly by the public sector, they have retained in all countries except Greece a certain amount of independence, either contracting independently with the public primary care services and public insurance organizations, or entering into such contracts through their medical associations.

As mentioned above, the system of health care delivery does not seem to make much difference to the level of health of the population, systems such as the fragmented one in the Federal Republic of Germany seeming to work in their own context, with the result that health indicators are high in that country, just as well as the more organized or centrally planned systems. The system – and particularly whether or not services are free at the point of use – and the way in which physicians are reimbursed can and do, however, make a difference to the demand for health services and therefore the demand for medical manpower services. To take the example of specialist services, in the United Kingdom and in Denmark, patients are referred to a specialist through the general practitioner, who under this system is very much the key to demand for his colleagues' services. In other EEC countries, the patient can present himself directly to the specialist for treatment.

Physicians paid on a fee-for-service basis obviously have more financial incentive to initiate demand for services than those paid on a salaried or per capita basis. Similarly, the incentive to refer a patient to another colleague, thus creating more demand for medical services, can also be affected by the method of payment.

All the EEC countries have public and private sectors existing side by side, although in the United Kingdom and Denmark for example, the private sector is only small. This can lead patients to make use of both sectors for the same incidence of illness, and also makes medical manpower planning more difficult.

3.3 Health Care Expenditure

From Table 3, the data for which are taken from the study by the Organization for Economic Co-operation and Development referred to earlier, it can be seen that there are large variations in per capita expenditure on medical care in the EEC region. These variations do not seem to be based entirely on the level of economic development, although the southern European countries and Ireland do seem to spend much less per capita than the northern European countries. Similarly, the variations do not seem to be closely related to a particular system of health care delivery, Belgium and the United Kingdom for example, which are at opposite ends of the scale with regard to their type of delivery system, having about the same level of spending.

Table 3. Per capita expenditure on medical care, 1982 (from [14])

Country	Per capita expenditure on health (US Dollar at current (1982) exchange rates)
Federal Republic of Germany	874
France	931
Italy	441
Netherlands	836
Belgium	534
Luxembourg	601
United Kingdom	508
Ireland	436
Denmark	746
Greece	187
Spain	302
Portugal	132

International comparisons of this nature are notoriously difficult because of a frequent lack of comparability in the data, and the above-mentioned study points out that no significance should be attached to small variations between countries. Even amongst the northern European states, however, there are very considerable differences.

Table 4 indicates total and public expenditure on health as a proportion of gross domestic product (GDP) between 1960 and 1980. Again, there is a clear difference between the northern and the southern member states. It is interesting to note that the countries with the largest public sectors (United Kingdom and Denmark) do not show comparatively high public expenditure on health.

The large increases in health expenditure occurred in the 1960s and early 1970s. In all countries of the EEC region, with the possible exception of Greece, where an attempt is being made to implement a new system, measures are being taken for cost containment in health care (29). Some of these measures are quite strong, including restricting access to services and introducing or increasing user payments.

3.4 Economic Growth

The world economic crisis following the increase in oil prices in the mid-1970s naturally affected the European region. In contrast to the rapid growth of the 1950s and 1960s, the EEC countries have been faced over the last decade with rising unemployment, high inflation, low growth, no economic growth or, in some cases, even a decline in GNP.

Although there have been signs of improvement, with a gradual deceleration of inflation rates since about 1980, annual growth rates are still rather low. The forecast growth rates for 1986 are a low of 1% for Greece, around 2% or less for Belgium, France, Luxembourg, the Netherlands and the United Kingdom, and a high of 3.5% for the Federal Republic of Germany (30).

Table 4. Share of expenditure on health in national expenditure, 1960–1982 (from [14])

Country	Total expenditure on health as % of GDP 1960	1970	1980	1982	Public expenditure on health as % of GDP 1960	1970	1980	1982
Federal Republic of Germany	4.8	5.6	6.1	8.2	3.2	4.2	6.5	6.6
France	4.3	6.1	8.5	9.3	2.5	4.3	6.1	6.6
Italy	3.9	5.5	6.8	7.2	3.2	4.8	6.0	6.1
Netherlands	3.9	6.0	8.3	8.7	1.3	5.1	6.5	6.9
Belgium	3.4	4.1	6.3	6.2	2.1	3.5	5.5	5.8
Luxembourg	–	4.9	6.6	7.4	–	–	6.5	6.6
United Kingdom	3.9	4.5	5.8	5.9	3.4	3.9	5.2	5.2
Ireland	4.0	5.6	8.7	8.2	3.0	4.3	8.1	7.7
Denmark	3.6	6.1	6.8	6.8	3.2	5.2	5.8	5.9
Greece	2.9	3.9	4.2	4.4	1.7	2.2	3.5	3.4
Spain	–	4.1	5.9	6.3	–	2.3	4.3	4.6
Portugal	–	–	6.1	5.7	0.9	1.9	4.2	4.0

Although inflation rates have fallen, except in Greece, to between about 2% and 8%, unemployment rates are still at levels ranging from about 8% to 17%. Unemployment has become a major social problem, for which there seems to be no quick and easy remedy.

Public debt has increased to hitherto unkown proportions in many of the EEC countries, accounting for over 100% of CDP in Belgium and Ireland, for example, and almost the same proportion in Italy.

4 Where Do the Above Trends Lead?

The expansion of the health sector in all countries of the EEC region is abundantly clear, and there is a very real danger that this is snowballing into a situation which can only be halted by very unpopular measures.

Advances in medical technology have made hitherto unheard-of treatment possible, while vast improvements in communications have meant that such high-technology treatment becomes quickly known through the news media, and is naturally demanded by patients and their relatives. Most of this high-technology treatment, however, is extremely expensive. Obviously, scientists cannot be expected to halt their search for new methods to alleviate human suffering, nor can medical personnel be expected not to utilize such methods to improve their work. Heart transplants, which were not so long ago a sensation, are much more commonplace, and the artificial heart is perhaps only one more step along this road of technical advances.

In some cases, advances in preserving life technical means have led to what can only be described as inhuman situations in which great suffering is prolonged. Particularly in some forms of cancer, the effects of the treatment can often be far worse than the symptoms of the disease itself (31).

The rapid expansion in medical manpower throughout the region has also led to increased costs. Apart from the salaries which must be paid to medical manpower and the pressure for high-technology treatment mentioned above, there is substantial evidence showing that an increase in doctors leads to an increase in consultations and in services authorized, such as X-rays and drugs (32).

The supply of medical manpower has expanded most rapidly in the hospital services. At the same time, hospitalization rates have been increasing in all the EEC countries. It can be seen from Table 5 that this increase has been quite considerable in many countries, particularly in France.

Although this can be partly explained by the aging of the population and the greater need of the elderly for health services, it is also a manifestation of the snowballing effect in the demand for health services.

In some cases, this explosion in the health sector has even been detrimental to health, notably with regard to the use of drugs. It has become a common practice to choose drugs to deal with social and psychological problems, and the overprescribing of psychoactive drugs, especially to women and old people, is a serious component of this problem (33).

Even the political environment can be conductive to an expanding health sector. More democratic procedures, which frequently involve greater decentralization of authority and participation of the community in decision-making, can lead to demands for the provision of expensive services at lower levels of administration. Each municipality would like to

Table 5. Number of persons hospitalized per 1000 population, 1971 and 1981 (from [14])

Country	Hospital admission rates per 1000 population 1971	1981
Federal Republic of Germany	150	181
France	79	120
Italy	137	158
Netherlands	101	118
Belgium	97	139
Luxembourg	139	170
United Kingdom	116	127
Ireland	132	176
Denmark	149	182
Greece	108	118

have its own full complement of services, and local politicians with an eye to the next elections can easily fall prey to persuasion from vociferous groups of either professionals or the public. A population which has learnt to organize itself effectively can sometimes impose certain developments, against the advice of specialists. An example of this way the experience concerning the demand for scanners in some areas of the United Kingdom, where in the face of decisions by certain authorities not to make such an investment, local people collected money to buy scanners, leaving the authorities to run them.

Although there have been some attempts to restrict the intake of medical students, these have not always been successful and have rarely been related to the expected needs for medical manpower. Systems such as that in Belgium, where university financing is related to student intake, have made universities loath to lose their numerical strength. The picture is also complicated by conflicting interests in the medical profession, with consultants demanding an increase in junior posts to ensure sufficient assistant, and junior doctors pressing for an increase in senior positions to expand their career prospects (34).

Consequently, the number of physicians unemployed is increasing, as is the length of unemployment. In Denmark, for example, if demand does not increase considerably or if there is no limitation on the supply of physicians, approximately 3000 doctors will become unemployed in the next 10 years.

The pressure on medical education and training facilities is increasing as the universities and training hospitals also feel the impact of the economic crisis. In some countries, this is already having a detrimental effect on the quality of medical graduates, and the situation can be expected to worsen unless measures are taken. As the national paper for Italy pointed out, there already exists a great mass of recently graduated physicians who have had inadequate practical training.

The increase in the number of specialists and the consequent use of their services for non-specialised treatment are impoverishing the scope for general practice. Similarly, the oversupply of physicians as a whole and their consequent engagement in activities which could be competently carried out by other health personnel are retarding the development of a more gratifying role for personnel such as nurses, for example.

This burgeoning of medical manpower is taking place in a situation in which medical manpower planning seems to be the exception rather than the rule. Bernard and Pendreigh have used terms such as "perceived shortage" and "common wisdom" as an indication of the essentially subjective nature of manpower calculations (35).

The demand for health manpower continues to be looked at in separate categories of physicians, nurses, etc. rather than with in a health-team framework, despite the fact that, as pointed out in the British paper, research has shown that opportunities for substitution between different inputs to medical care are considerable. This continued compartmentalisation does not allow for the examination of real alternatives and simply shores up the status quo.

The national papers of Denmark and Greece specifically point out that in those countries there is no medical audit system or provision for peer review. Although medical personnel are expensive professionals both in terms of the cost of their training and their remuneration, comparatively little is being done to investigate what they are offering with regard to effectiveness and efficiency. Despite protestations of belief in the principles of equity, there has been little examination of the ways in which medical manpower could be instrumental in achieving greater equity, and there is a very real danger that present inequities will continue or increase.

With unlimited resources, there would be no reason for not having a hospital in every community, a doctor's surgery on every street and transplants for every patient suitable for such treatment. Resources are not unlimited, however, and the health sector is not alone in making demands on scarce resources. There are still population groups living in poverty, and social security systems are experiencing difficulties in meeting future pension needs. Special groups, albeit small in number, need help with severe problems such as drug addiction, child abuse, etc. As seen above, large groups of the EEC population are unemployed, and this is particularly serious amongst the young. In other words, large sections of the population are being deprived of their fundemantal rights to participate in social and economic life, and to develop to the full their talents and personalities, whilst at the same time a large proportion of resources is being spent on health services which either benefit very small groups of the population or are of uncertain value in improving the level of health.

5 What Can Be Done?

The picture looks quite sombre. If it is to be ameliorated, some quite strong measures will need to be taken, and to be taken quickly.

5.1 Health for All by the Year 2000

At the 30th session of the WHO European Regional Committe in 1980, the representatives of member states approved their first common health policy (36). This strategy sets out fundamental requirements which must be fulfilled if people are to be healthy, and defines improvements in health that could be achieved by the year 2000. It calls for fundamental changes in countries' health development, involving emphasis on health promotion and disease prevention, as well as on the role of the individual, families and the community, and advocates primary care as the major approach to the delivery of health services.

The EEC countries have already subscribed to this strategy, but if more than lip-service is to be paid to it. considerable administrative and organizational changes will be needed, and these will have a direct impact on medical manpower planning.

5.2 Changes in Planning

The HFA 2000 strategy is multisectoral. However, it is clear from the above that planning for health in the countries of the EEC region is rarely multisectoral.

Planning for health must therefore become an *integrated part of overall development planning*, and can no longer be carried out on a purely sectoral basis. The way in which this is achieved will obviously vary as the system of development planning varies among the countries of the region, from countries which formulate comprehensive plans to those in which such state guidance is minimal. The integration of health planning into development planning means not only taking a multisectoral approach to health but also much more explicit priority setting between sectors of development. When there are difficult decisions to be taken as there are now, decision-making must perforce be more explicit. The general public must be made aware that investment in health means less investment for housing, roads, education, etc.

The first step will need to be the *planning of the planning process itself*, which includes the training of planners. Most of the EEC countries have some sort of National Health Council which advises the responsible minister on health policy. On the whole, however, if one judges by their membership, they appear to be sectorally orientated. WHO has suggested that *multisectoral National Health Councils* would be conducive to the radical change in planning which is needed (37).

It may be useful to consider where health planners are to be situated in the planning process. Can they continue to be situated only in Ministries of Health or National Health Councils, or does the Ministry of Health need to deplay some of its planners within ministries responsible for other sectors such as industry, agriculture, housing, public works, etc.?

5.3 Changes in the System of Health Services Delivery

Target 26 of the European strategy for HFA 2000 is a *system based on primary health care* and supported by secondary and tertiary care. This calls for effective legislation, regulations and plans. It is not only a question of national governments' adopting such a policy and outlining the appropriate guidelines. Particularly in those EEC countries where the system is extremely decentralised or even fragmented, this means that the insurance funds and the public itself must realize the necessity of this change in the structure of the delivery of health services. They will have to look not only at the division between primary, secondary and tertiary care but also at the *position and role of the physician within the health care team.* The function of every member of the health team, whether in hospital or extramural care, will need to be seen in relation to that of each of his colleagues, and possibilities for substitution will need to be considered, for the achievement of greater effectiveness and efficiency.

More provision for part-time employment in the health services must be considered, for the purpose of facilitating greater female participation and perhaps early part-time retirement.

5.4 Medial Education

Such a shift in the health system will need *changes in the education and training of physicians,* and if more rapid results are to be obtained, provisions for the *retraining of some physicians.* The universities, medical associations and manpower planners will need to give this the highest priority.

If medical education is to be relevant, more needs to be known, as mentioned above, about the *present and expected "job description" of the physician, and the effectiveness and efficiency of medical activities.* The "job description" or role of the physician will necessarily need to be looked at from a national perspective, but with regard to effectiveness and efficiency, co-operation and pooling of information at the Community level would also be valuable.

It has been pointed out that restriction of access to higher education is a sensitive subject which can have strong political connotations, Belgium in particular having so far found it impossible to enforce a *numerus clausus* system. The younger generation must be made fully aware, however, that *6–12 years of hard study may very well lead to unemployment.* It is of little use to inform parents and young people in the last year of secondary school of the possible employment difficulties ahead. At that stage, many young people have already formed their own ideas about their future. They *need to be informed at a much younger age.*

Where this is not a political problem, restriction of access to medical education seems unavoidable. Manpower studies forecasting the possible extent of medical unemployment will need to be discussed publicly, and their results published in an easily understood form, if such restrictions are to be accepted by the general public. The members of the scientific community cannot continue to discuss the question of medical education among themselves.

Particular attention will need to be given to the assessment of expected demand for specialists, both in relation to the desired changes in the structure of health services and in view of demographic developments, the expansion of family planning services and new illness patterns, i.e. drug addiction, iatrogenic illness and sexually transmitted diseases. In other words, medical manpower planners will need to think more in terms of measuring medical activities or functions within the framework of new health service delivery systems, rather than simply in terms of physician-population ratios on the basis of extrapolations of existing systems.

Continuing increases in the level of female participation in medical education may also become extremely important, and the possible consequences of this need to be given particular attention.

5.5 *Medical Sociology*

Society and the framework within in which health care, and therefore the role of medical manpower, must be seen have been undergoing rapid changes during the twentieth century. Today's medical graduates will go out into a society which is already quite different in some respects from that faced by their colleagues of even 10 years ago, and which can be expected to have changed again over the next decade or two.

Medical sociology has not been developed to the same extent in all EEC member countries. The training and role of the physician must be seen in the context of a changing family unit (aging family members, changing sex roles within the family, smaller family units, including single-member families, etc.); in the context of the demand by women for a different attitude towards health care, particularly as this affects their reproductive role; in the face of high unemployment rates and their impact on health; and with regard to new life-styles.

5.6 *Participation in the Instigation of Change*

The necessary changes will not come about by wishful thinking or even government exhortation. Various groups must be rapidly and vigorously activated.

First and foremost, there is a need for *community participation,* which entails broad public education through the *mass media.* The average citizen – the man in the street – must be made aware of the complexity of the health question, of the cost of health services and what this means in terms of alternative patterns of development, and of his indivual responsibility of his own health. It is interesting in this respect that one of the newest members of the Community, Portugal, in addition to declaring the citizen's "right" to health, has also tried to list his "responsibilities".

The ethical problems which have become more acute owing to the advances in medical technology mentioned above cannot be a matter for the medical profession alone, nor can they be solved by technocrats. Only society itself can make the difficult ethical decisions involved in setting priorities and allocating resources. To do this with any degree of responsibility, the public must be informed.

Secondly, the *medical associations,* both nationally and internationally, need to play a more active role. Obviously, they cannot be expected to behave entirely altruistically, without trying to protect the interests of their members, which sometimes conflict with those of their patients, particularly as taxpayers. No real change can be effected, however, without the agreement of the medical profession. There is a need, therefore, for the medical profession itself to re-examine its role and position in a changing society.

The profession also needs to re-examine its members employment prospects, and to take a position on this. The Danish experience, described in the Danish national paper, of restricting overtime in order to create new positions is a case in point. Such position-taking can be painful, but it is going to be unavoidable.

The *medical schools and university hospitals* will also need to be active in reassesing their own orientation. It is clear from the national papers in this study that medical education is not sufficiently orientated toward producing top-quality doctors for primary care.

Only when the academic world bestows the same esteem on "especialists" in primary care as on specialists in other fields can primary care achieve prestige in the eyes of the public.

The type of doctor needed for a primary care system with a multisectoral approach to health care according to which the patient is an active participant is different from the doctor who, with his superior professional knowledge, paternalistically directs and guides his grateful flock. The medical schools as centres of research, in co-operation with the medical associations, can take the lead in *redefining the role of the primary care physician and consequently of the specialists* who will be called upon to provide the back-up services for a new type of primary care.

The *trade unions* in EEC countries have not always been very active in the health field, apart from their concern mainly for safety precautions in the workplace and compensation for work-related disabilities. A multisectoral approach to health presupposes not only the examination of health conditions in the workplace as these have traditionally been defined but also an assessment of methods of production and the health impact of unemployment. The vast majority of the labour force in the EEC countries are wage and salary earners, and their unions can act as two-way channels of communication, assisting in the dissemination of information to their members and participating in the public discussion on the redifinition of the role of the health services system and of medical manpower in that system.

Representatives of *special groups* such as feminist organizations and pensioners will need to play a similar role. The voices of these two population groups are particularly important, given the impact of extramural health care on women as the main informal care-givers, and the importance of pensioners as increasingly heavy users of the health services.

5.7 Information and Research

The lack of a sufficient information background for medical manpower planning is obvious from the national papers and was particularly emphasised in the British paper. In parts of the EEC region, particularly the southern countries, even quite basic statistics are lacking. National governments will need to set the wheels in motion for the conpilation of the necessary data and for the channelling of funds for research into the areas of concern mentioned above.

Some of the areas which will need high priority are those concerning "models" of health service delivery and the potentiality for input substitutions; the further development of indicators to assess the quality of medical services and their impact on health status; means of achieving greater equity; and methods of ensuring meaningful participation by patients and public.

The EEC can play a valuable role in assisting in the pooling of research efforts and in bringing the results of this research to the attention of policy-makers.

References

1. Basic Documents. WHO, twenty-sixth edition, 1976, p 1
2. Mangerical process for national health development. WHO, Geneva, 1981, p 9
3. Hall TL, Mejia A (eds) Health manpower planning – prinicples, methods, issues. WHO, Geneva, 1978
4. Fuchs V (ed) Essays in the economics of health and medical care. National Bureau of Economic Research, New York, 1972
5. Abel-Smith B, Maynard A (1979) The organization, financing and cost of health care in the European Community. Social Policy Series, Commission of the European Community, Brüssel
6. Abel-Smith, B (1984) in van der Werff A (ed) Public Administration and health services in Western Europe. European Institute of Public Administration, Maastricht
7. Measurement of levels of health. WHO, Regional Office for Europe, Copenhagen, 1979, p 25
8. Falk N, Lee J (1978) Planning the social services. Saxon House, Farnborough
9. Forsyth G, Logan RF (1960) The demand for medical care. Nuffield Provincial Hospital Trust, London
10. Health planning-problems of concept and method. CENDES in cooperation with the Pan American Sanitary Bureau, Scientific Publication No. 111, Washington, 1965
11. Oncu A (1982) quoted in Hǫiberg A (ed) Women and the world of work. Plenum Press, New York London, p 8
12. Commission of the European Communities (1984) Recognition of diplomas and professional qualifications. European File, 13/84, August-September, 1984, p 7
13. Statistical tables relating to the migration of doctors in the community form 1977 to 1983. Commission of the European Communities III D/1098/1/82EN, Brussels, 5.2.1985
14. Measuring health care 1960–1983 – Expenditure, costs and performance. OECD, Paris, 1985
15. The uses of epidermiology in the study of the elderly. WHO Technical Report Series 706, Geneva, 1984, p 13
16. Ibid. p 20
17. Prims AV (1984) Public administration and health services in Belgium. In: van de Werff A (ed) Public administration and health services in Western Europe, vol. II, European Institute of Public Administration, Maastricht
18. ibid. p 18
19. Blanpain JE (1984) The health services system in Belgium. In: Pannenborg CO, van der Werff A, Hirsch GB, Barnard K (eds) Reorienting health systems – application of a systems approach. Nato Conference Series II, vol 15, Plenum Press, New York London, p 251
20. Rossing N: Public administration and health services in Denmark. In: European Institute of Public Administration, op. cit., p 28
21. Roualt J: Public administration and health services in France. In: European Institute of Public Administration, cp. cit.
22. Affeld D: Public administration and health services in the Federal Republic of Germany. In: European Institute of Public Administration, op. cit.
23. Ritsatakis A: Public administration and health services in Greece. In: European Institute of Public Administration, op. cit.
24. Paderni S, Piergentili P: Public administration and health services in Italy. In: European Institute of Public Administration, op. cit.
25. Dwyer JO: Public administration and health services in Ireland. In: European Institute of Public Administration, op. cit.
26. Abel-Smith B, Graham CF: Public administration and health services in England. In: European Institute of Public Administration, op. cit.

27. Hemmer CA: Public administration and health services in Luxembourg. In: European Institute of Public Administration, op. cit.
28. van der Heuvel R, Roscam Abbing H: Public administration and the health services in the Netherlands. In: European Institute of Public Administration, op. cit.
29. Abel-Smith B (1984) Cost containment in health care – a study of 12 European countries 1977–1983. Occasional Papers in Social Administration, No. 73, Bedford Square Press, NCVC, London
30. European Economy. Commission of the European Community, Directorate General for Economic and Financial Affairs, Supplement A, No. 10, Oct 1985
31. Health care in a changing setting: the U.K. experience. CIBA Foundation Symposium 43, Elsevier/Excerpta Medica/North Holland, Amsterdam Oxford New York, 1976, p 146
32. Abel-Smith (1984) op. cit., p 8
33. Targets for health for all. WHO, Regional Office for Europe, Copenhagen, 1985, p 71
34. Barnard K, Pendreigh D: The health services system of the United Kingdom. In: Nato Conference Series (1984) op. cit.
35. ibid. p 324
36. WHO (1985) op. cit.
37. i) Broad programming as part of the managerial process for national health development, WHO, Geneva, December 1981
    ii) Managerial process for national health development. WHO, Geneva, 1981

GPSR Compliance

The European Union's (EU) General Product Safety Regulation (GPSR) is a set of rules that requires consumer products to be safe and our obligations to ensure this.

If you have any concerns about our products, you can contact us on ProductSafety@springernature.com

In case Publisher is established outside the EU, the EU authorized representative is:

Springer Nature Customer Service Center GmbH
Europaplatz 3
69115 Heidelberg, Germany

Batch number: 10704763

Printed by Printforce, the Netherlands